Skin: Discourse on Emerging Science and Techniques

CLINICS IN PLASTIC SURGERY

www.plasticsurgery.theclinics.com

January 2012 • Volume 39 • Number 1

SAUNDERS an imprint of ELSEVIER, Inc.

W.B. SAUNDERS COMPANY
A Division of Elsevier Inc.

1600 John F. Kennedy Boulevard • Suite 1800 • Philadelphia, Pennsylvania 19103-2899

http://www.theclinics.com

CLINICS IN PLASTIC SURGERY Volume 39, Number 1
January 2012 ISSN 0094-1298, ISBN-13: 978-1-4557-3919-6

Editor: Joanne Husovski

Clinics in Plastic Surgery (ISSN 0094-1298) is published quarterly by Elsevier Inc., 360 Park Avenue South, New York, NY 10010-1710. Months of issue are January, April, July, and October. Business and Editorial Offices: 1600 John F. Kennedy Blvd., Suite 1800, Philadelphia, PA 19103-2899. Periodicals postage paid at New York, NY and additional mailing offices. Subscription prices are $448.00 per year for US individuals, $666.00 per year for US institutions, $221.00 per year for US students and residents, $509.00 per year for Canadian individuals, $779.00 per year for Canadian institutions, $578.00 per year for international individuals, $779.00 per year for international institutions, and $279.00 per year for Canadian and foreign students/residents. To receive student/resident rate, orders must be accompanied by name of affiliated institution, date of term, and the *signature* of program/residency coordinator on institution letterhead. Orders will be billed at individual rate until proof of status is received. Foreign air speed delivery is included in all *Clinics* subscription prices. All prices are subject to change without notice. **POSTMASTER:** Send address changes to *Clinics in Plastic Surgery*, Elsevier Health Sciences Division, Subscription Customer Service, 3251 Riverport Lane, Maryland Heights, MO 63043. **Customer Service: 1-800-654-2452 (US and Canada). From outside of the United States and Canada, call 314-447-8871. Fax: 314-447-8029. E-mail: JournalsCustomerService-usa@elsevier.com (for print support); JournalsOnlineSupport-usa@elsevier.com (for online support).**

Reprints. For copies of 100 or more of articles in this publication, please contact the Commercial Reprints Department, Elsevier Inc., 360 Park Avenue South, New York, New York 10010-1710. Tel.: (+1) 212-633-3812; Fax: (+1) 212-462-1935; E-mail: reprints@elsevier.com.

Clinics in Plastic Surgery is covered in *Current Contents, EMBASE/Excerpta Medica, Science Citation Index, MEDLINE/PubMed (Index Medicus), ASCA,* and *ISI/BIOMED.*

Printed and bound by CPI Group (UK) Ltd, Croydon, CR0 4YY

Transferred to Digital Print 2012

Contributors

AUTHORS

THOMAS BLATT
R&D, Beiersdorf, Hamburg, Germany

HUI CHEN
Department of Burns, Beijing Jishuitan Hospital, Beijing, People's Republic of China

XIN CHEN
Department of Burns, Beijing Jishuitan Hospital, Beijing, People's Republic of China

ERIC A. GANTWERKER, MD
Resident Physician, Department of Otolaryngology–Head and Neck Surgery, University of Cincinnati and Cincinnati Children's Hospital Medical Center, Cincinnati, Ohio

P.M. GEARY
Department of Plastic Surgery, Salisbury District Hospital, Odstock Centre for Burns and Plastic Surgery, Salisbury District Hospital, Odstock, Salisbury, Wiltshire, United Kingdom

FLORIAN GROEBER
Department of Cell and Tissue Engineering, Fraunhofer-Institute for Interfacial Engineering and Biotechnology (IGB); Institute for Interfacial Engineering, Stuttgart, Germany

MARTINA HAMPEL
Department of Cell and Tissue Engineering, Fraunhofer-Institute for Interfacial Engineering and Biotechnology (IGB); Institute for Interfacial Engineering, Stuttgart, Germany

SVENJA HINDERER
Department of Cell and Tissue Engineering, Fraunhofer-Institute for Interfacial Engineering and Biotechnology (IGB), Stuttgart; Faculty of Medicine, Eberhard Karls University Tübingen, Germany

MONIKA HOLEITER
Department of Cell and Tissue Engineering, Fraunhofer-Institute for Interfacial Engineering and Biotechnology (IGB), Stuttgart; Faculty of Medicine, Eberhard Karls University Tübingen, Germany

DAVID B. HOM, MD
Professor, Division of Facial Plastic and Reconstructive Surgery, Division of Facial Plastic and Reconstructive Surgery, Department of Otolaryngology–Head and Neck Surgery, University of Cincinnati and Cincinnati Children's Hospital Medical Center, Cincinnati, Ohio

SOEREN JASPERS
R&D, Beiersdorf, Hamburg, Germany

JOSEF A. KÄS
Division of Soft Matter Physics, Department of Physics, University of Leipzig, Leipzig, Germany

JEAN KRUTMANN
Institut für Umweltmedizinische Forschung (IUF) at the Heinrich-Heine-University, Düsseldorf gGmbH, Düsseldorf, Germany

THOMAS KUEPER
R&D, Beiersdorf, Hamburg, Germany

J. LABAT-ROBERT
Laboratoire de Recherche Ophtalmologique, Université Paris-5, Paris, France

J.K.G. LAITUNG
Department of Plastic and Reconstructive Surgery, Royal Preston Hospital, Preston, Lancashire, United Kingdom

ANKE MALSEN
R&D, Beiersdorf, Hamburg, Germany

GESA MUHR
R&D, Beiersdorf, Hamburg, Germany

A.-M. ROBERT
Laboratoire de Recherche Ophtalmologique,
Université Paris-5, Paris, France

L. ROBERT
Laboratoire de Recherche Ophtalmologique,
Université Paris-5, Paris, France

KATJA SCHENKE-LAYLAND
Department of Cell and Tissue Engineering,
Fraunhofer-Institute for Interfacial Engineering
and Biotechnology (IGB), Stuttgart; Faculty of
Medicine, Eberhard Karls University Tübingen,
Germany

CHRISTIAN SCHULZE
Division of Soft Matter Physics, Department
of Physics, University of Leipzig, Leipzig; R&D,
Beiersdorf, Hamburg, Germany

K. SENARATH-YAPA
Department of Plastic and Reconstructive
Surgery, Royal Preston Hospital, Preston,
Lancashire, United Kingdom

S.H.A. SHAH
Department of Plastic and Reconstructive
Surgery, Royal Preston Hospital, Preston,
Lancashire, United Kingdom

E. TIERNAN
Department of Plastic Surgery, Salisbury
District Hospital, Odstock Centre for Burns
and Plastic Surgery, Salisbury District Hospital,
Odstock, Salisbury, Wiltshire, United Kingdom

R.A.J. WAIN
Department of Plastic and Reconstructive
Surgery, Royal Preston Hospital, Preston,
Lancashire, United Kingdom

HORST WENCK
R&D, Beiersdorf, Hamburg, Germany

FRANZISKA WETZEL
Division of Soft Matter Physics, Department of
Physics, University of Leipzig, Leipzig, Germany

KLAUS-PETER WITTERN
R&D, Beiersdorf, Hamburg, Germany

FIONA WOOD
Burns Service of Western Australia, Burn Injury
Research Unit, University of Western Australia,
McComb Research Foundation, Western
Australia

GUOAN ZHANG
Department of Burns, Beijing Jishuitan
Hospital, Beijing, People's Republic of China

Contents

Skin is the most voluminous organ of the body. It assumes several important phys-iological functions and represents also a "social interface" between an individual and other members of society. This is the main reason its age-dependent modifications are in the forefront of dermatological research and of the "anti-aging" cosmetic in-dustry. Here we concentrate on some aspects only of skin aging, as far as the cel-lular and extracellular matrix components of skin are concerned. Most well studied mechanisms of skin aging can be situated at the postgenetic level, both epigenetic and post-translational mechanisms being involved. Some of these mechanisms will be reviewed as well as the capacity of fucose- and rhamnose-rich oligo- and poly-saccharides (FROP and RROP) to counteract several of the mechanisms involved in skin aging.

Changes in mechanical properties are an essential characteristic of the aging pro-cess of human skin. Previous studies attribute these changes predominantly to the altered collagen and elastin organization and density of the extracellular matrix. Here, we show that individual dermal fibroblasts also exhibit a significant increase in stiffness during aging in vivo. With the laser-based optical cell stretcher we exam-ined the viscoelastic biomechanics of dermal fibroblasts isolated from 14 human do-nors aged 27 to 80. Increasing age was clearly accompanied by a stiffening of the investigated cells. We found that fibroblasts from old donors exhibited an increase in rigidity of ~60% with respect to cells of the youngest donors. A FACS analysis of the content of the cytoskeletal polymers shows a shift from monomeric G-actin to polymerized, filamentous F-actin, but no significant changes in the vimentin and microtubule content. The rheological analysis of fibroblast-populated collagen gels demonstrates that cell stiffening directly results in altered viscoelastic proper-ties of the collagen matrix. These results identify a new mechanism that may contrib-ute to the age-related impairment of elastic properties in human skin. The altered mechanical behavior might influence cell functions involving the cytoskeleton, such as contractility, motility, and proliferation, which are essential for reorganization of the extracellular matrix.

Each one of us is a self-organizing mass of multiple cell types. From fertilization of the embryo our tissue structures develop until an adult morphology is achieved. At that point our capacity for self-organization is directed to maintaining that mor-phology in the face of the insults of our daily life and the processes of aging. When a given insult overwhelms our capacity to repair by regeneration the result is scar repair.

Significant progress has been made over the years in the development of in vitro-engineered substitutes that mimic human skin, either to be used as grafts for the replacement of lost skin or for the establishment of human-based in vitro skin models. This review summarizes these advances in in vivo and in vitro applications of tissue-engineered skin. We further highlight novel efforts in the design of complex disease-in-a-dish models for studies ranging from disease etiology to drug development and screening.

Current research on the complex interplay between the microbiota, the barrier function and the innate immune system of the skin indicates that the skin's microbiota have a beneficial role, much like that of the gut microflora. As a consequence, interest in strategies beyond antibiotica that allow a more selective modulation of the skin microflora is constantly growing. This review will briefly summarize our current understanding of the cutaneous microbiota and summarize existing information on pre- and probiotic strategies for skin.

Large, full-thickness calvarial defects present a series of significant reconstructive challenges involving a range of techniques, including local and free flaps. Occasionally these conventional methods may not be possible due to technical, or patient, factors. Artificial dermis is already widely used in burns surgery and is increasing in oncological reconstruction. We believe that artificial dermis coupled with split-thickness skin grafting provides an excellent option for closure of these defects when other techniques are not appropriate.

The task of managing an open wound complicated by exposed bony structures underneath is difficult, if not challenging. We have instituted a method of managing the problems in stages using an artificial dermis and skin grafting technique in 17 wounds in 15 individuals from Sept. 2006 to Feb. 2009. While all wounds were noted to assume aberrant healing processes, the majority of involved bony structures were devoid of periosteal covering compounded by various degrees of infection. Of 15 incidents, mechanical trauma was responsible for 10, chemical burns for two and electrical burns for two patients. A chronic non-healing ulcer with exposed bone formed in an old burn scar accounted for the remaining one. The regimen of surgical management consisted of initial debridement, the coverage of the resultant wound with an artificial dermis and a partial-thickness skin grafted over this dermis-like structure grown with granulation tissues. Complete wound healing was attained in 15 out of 17 with outstanding cosmetic and minimal donor-site morbidity. Despite initial failure encountered in two, the morbidities noted were low. It is especially useful in large defects that usually require flaps for coverage.

Management of Split Skin Graft Donor Sites–Results of a National Survey   77

P.M. Geary and E. Tiernan

The authors wished to obtain a 'snapshot' of the range of practice in the management of split skin graft donor sites in the British Isles. Material/Methods Questionnaires were sent to all British consultants and locum consultant plastic surgeons on July 1, 2006. Of the 357 questionnaires, 279 were returned (a response rate of 78%). Results Alginates were the most popular dressings, especially in adult donor sites – first choice for 167 respondents (60%). Adhesive fabrics were less popular – first choice for small adult donor areas for 46 respondents (16%). Plastic film dressings and Biobrane were even less popular – being the first choice for small and large donor areas, respectively, in children (for approximately 5% of respondents). Ten percent of respondents said they avoid paraffin gauze and another 10% avoid plastic film dressings in all cases. Five percent avoid hydrocolloid and another 5% avoid adhesive fabric in all cases. Conclusion on the basis of these results, the authors feel that any future study of donor-site dressings should incorporate the most commonly used dressing (alginate) as a control.

Skin: Histology and Physiology of Wound Healing   85

Eric A. Gantwerker and David B. Hom

It is important to understand the histology and physiology of skin for the prediction and optimization of wound healing. Optimal postoperative wound healing to minimize scarring entails minimizing local, systemic, and environmental factors that lead to poor wound healing. Keeping the wound clean and moist, minimizing trauma, and infection are the local wound tenets. Systemic tenets include minimizing medications that inhibit processes of wound healing, maintaining adequate nutrition, pain palliation, UV protection, and smoking cessation. This article presents the dynamic process of wound healing and the basic tenets to minimize scarring.

Index   99

Clinics in Plastic Surgery

THE CLINICS ARE AVAILABLE ONLINE!

Access your subscription at:
www.theclinics.com

Publisher's Note

The compilation of articles in this issue is intended to share the broad array of clinical and scientific research underway on skin: its physiology, architecture, behavior, and the potential and challenges in engineering it from tissue and cells.

Top scientists, researchers, and clinicians from Europe, Australia, Asia, and the United States are represented in this selection of articles intended for plastic surgeons to follow the progress of new research and to make clinical use with the current state of the art of skin knowledge – aging, resurfacing, flaps, and regeneration.

"Every artist undresses his subject, whether human or still life. It is his business to find essences in surfaces, and what more attractive and challenging surface than the skin around a soul?"

—Richard Corliss - Writer

Clin Plastic Surg 39 (2012) ix
doi:10.1016/j.cps.2011.09.013

plasticsurgery.theclinics.com

Physiology of Skin Aging

L. Robert*, J. Labat-Robert, A.-M. Robert

KEYWORDS

- Skin • Aging • Fibroblasts • Keratinocytes
- Extracellular matrix • Elastases • Free radicals
- Maillard reaction • Receptors

INTRODUCTION

It is now largely accepted that aging is not "coded" in the genome although modifications of the coordination of gene functions are certainly involved. The hereditary genetic influences, put to about 25% a few decades ago, are now considered to represent no more than about 3%.[1] Evolution apparently did not care much about aging, perhaps to some extent indirectly since the Paleolithic because of the "grandmother" effect. Most well studied, reproducible mechanisms can be situated at the epigenetic and postsynthetic (post-translational) level.[2] Sirtuins, claimed to produce when stimulated an extension of lifespan, act clearly at the epigenetic level.[3,4] Those mechanisms shown to be involved in skin aging are also driven by epigenetic and post-translational mechanisms. Some of these processes will be described.

MECHANISMS OF SKIN AGING

The most conspicuous process is certainly the progressive loss of skin tissue. Measured by image-analytical techniques on skin biopsies taken at sun-protected sites (**Fig. 1**), skin loss amounts on the average to about 7% per decade with however large individual variations.[5] This loss of skin tissue, which underlies most of the easily noticed morphological modifications of the skin, can be attributed to several factors such as loss of cells and loss of extracellular matrix (ECM). Cell loss concerns both the epidermal and dermal layers. Loss of ECM is evident when histological skin sections from young and old individuals are compared. Loss of ECM is the result of cell loss, decreased biosynthetic capacity of remaining cells and to a progressive increase of matrix degrading enzymes.

Loss of Cells

Loss of cells is currently attributed to two distinct processes: slow-down of cell division because of telomere loss and exit of cells from the mitotic pool mediated by some antioncogenes through a "switch mechanism" enabling cells to quit the mitotic pool entering the senescent phenotype, escaping thus from malignancy.[6] This teleological presentation of the observed facts corresponds probably to a stress-mediated process of phenotypic switch. This process might well play an important role in the loss of mitotic cells as shown by our experiments, reproduced on **Fig. 2**. It is clear that the rate of loss of telomeres is slower than the loss of skin tissue. The difference, of about 3.5 fold in the two slopes shown on **Fig. 2**, is probably an indication of the importance of other mechanisms, such as the antioncogene mediated switch to the postmitotic phenotype. More recently, a third mechanism was described by McClintock et al.[7] These authors showed that progerin accumulates in skin during aging. Progerin is a dominant negative form of lamin A, a nuclear membrane protein which is produced in cells of young individuals affected by the Hutchinson-Gilford syndrome (progeria) and who die young

This article originally published in *Pathologie Biologie, 47 (2009), 336-341, Elsevier.*
Laboratoire de recherche ophtalmologique, université Paris-5, Hôtel-Dieu, 1, place du Parvis-Notre-Dame, 75181 Paris cedex 04, France
* Corresponding author.
E-mail address: lrobert5@wanadoo.fr

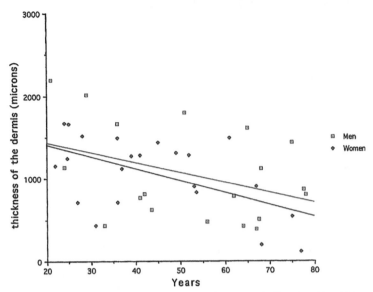

Fig. 1. Loss of human skin thickness with age. Abscissa: age in years. Ordinates: skin thickness in micrometers, measured by morphometry on fixed skin biopsies from a sun-protected site (*Data from* Branchet MC, Boisnic S, Francès C, et al. Skin thickness changes in normal aging skin. Gerontology 1990;36:28–35.).

(12–15 years) with cardiovascular symptoms. Ninety percent of these cases carry the LMNA G608G (CGC > CCT) mutation within exon 11 of LMNA. This mutation activates a splice donor site resulting in the production of truncated lamin

A designated progerin. The progressive accumulation of this molecular marker of cellular aging was achieved by the use of a specific antibody and immunolabeling of progerin in skin biopsies. Further studies will undoubtedly reveal the importance

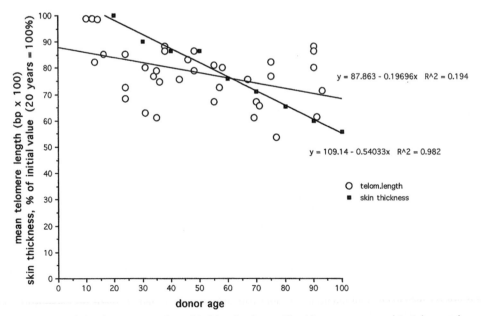

Fig. 2. Comparison of skin loss measured on skin biopsies (as on **Fig. 1.**): ■; as compared to telomere loss of skin fibroblasts: ○ (*From* Ravelojaona V, Robert AM, Robert L. Expression of senescence-associated b-galactosidase by human skin fibroblasts. Effect of advanced glycation end products and fucose- or rhamnose-rich polysaccharides. Arch Gerontol Geriatr 2009;48:151–4; with permission.).[34]

of this new biomarker of skin aging. Among the clinical symptoms in children affected by this rare disease is, among others the absence of subcutaneous adipose tissue which contributes to the senile appearence of the head and face of these children.

Increased Degradation of Skin-ECM

Among the early findings we made during our studies on aging of connective tissues, the most conspicuous was the progressive upregulation of elastase-type endopeptidase activity. This was first demonstrated on human aorta extracts devoid of atherosclerotic lesions.[8] As shown on **Fig. 3**, the elastase-type activity of aorta extracts increased exponentially with donor age. Similar findings were reported on mouse skin extracts, an exponential increase of elastase-type activity with

age, further potentialised by UV-radiation.[9] To our surprise, similar upregulation of elastase-type endopeptidase activity was seen when the determinations were carried out on successive passages of arterial smooth muscle cells or on human skin fibroblasts (**Fig. 3**). Although the mechanism of this intrinsic cellular phenomenon is not yet elucidated, epigenetic modifications increasing the expression of MMP-2 and MMP-9 coding genes are the most plausible.[10] There was a strong increase of elastase-type activity of vascular smooth muscle cell cultures in presence of athero-genic lipoproteins, LDL and VLDL. Lipid deposition in the skin, depending at least partially on the quality and quantity of dietary intake, may therefore represent an important factor for the regulation of skin proteolytic activity.

POSTSYNTHETIC MECHANISMS OF SKIN AGING
The Maillard Reaction

The importance of glycation for the aging of connective tissues was first convincingly demonstrated by the experiments of Verzar.[11] He showed that the tensile strength of tendons, essentially of collagen fibers, increased exponentially with age (**Fig. 4**). He correctly attributed this process to increasing crosslinking. Later it was shown that glycation by reducing sugars and related molecules is involved.[12] A great number of studies were published since these early observations on the production of advanced glycation end-products (AGE-products) and on their role in tissue aging.[13] We took up this subject during the last few years showing that in vitro prepared AGE-products could directly kill fibroblasts when added even at low concentrations to cultures.[14] As shown on **Table 1**, two of the AGE-products tested

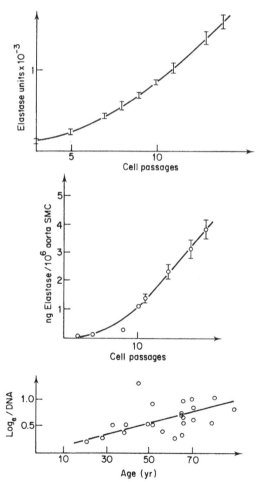

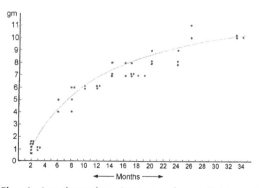

Fig. 4. Age-dependent increase of cross-linking of collagen fibers (rat tail tendon) attributed to the Maillard reaction (*Data from* Robert L. Fritz Verzar was born 120 years ago: his contribution to experimental gerontology through the collagen research as assessed after half a century. Arch Gerontol Geriatr 2006;43:13–43.).

Fig. 3. Increase of elastase-type endopeptidase activity in human aortas with age (*bottom*), with passage number in vascular smooth muscle cells (*middle graph*) and human skin fibroblasts (*upper graph*).

Table 1
Action of AGE-products on human skin fibroblasts

AGE Added	% Cell Death	Proliferation
Control	1553 = 100%	100%
Lysozyme–glucose 9.2 µM	+268	+100
BSA–Glc-Fe 0.41 µM	+369	–
Lysine–Glc 550 µM	+539	+565
Arg–Glc 550 µM	+263	+324

Cell death and cell proliferation were studied, both in % increase as compared to control (*Data from* Péterszegi G, Molinari J, Ravelojaona V, et al. Effect of advanced glycation end-products on cell proliferation and cell death. Pathol Biol 2006;54:396–404.).
Number of cells seeded: 4×10^4.

strongly increased cell death and also cell proliferation. AGE-products were also shown to increase elastase-type endopeptidase expression when added to human skin fibroblasts (**Fig. 5**). As AGE-products are derived not only from local production in tissues by glycation and glycoxydation but are also absorbed with dietary sources.[15] Their local concentration does certainly increase with time. Their role in the age-dependent increase of elastase-type endopeptidase production might therefore be important.

Proteolytic Production of Toxic Peptides

This process, progressively uncovered during the last decades, might well play an important role in tissue aging. Let us take as an exemple fibronectin (FN). We could show that its production is increasing with age.[16] The two chains of FN, composed of relatively compact subunits, are easily degraded by proteolytic enzymes, also shown to be upregulated during aging (**Fig. 3**). Several of the peptides released by proteases were shown to exhibit harmful effects: potentiation of malignant transformation, pro-inflammatory activity, proper proteolytic activity absent in the parent-molecule. One fragment of FN was shown to upregulate the biosynthesis of fibronectin.[17] Similar processes were shown to be produced by degradation products of other ECM macromolecules such as elastin peptides. Although these mechanisms are rather widespread in tissues, their contribution to age-dependent modifications has still to be quantitatively evaluated.

Loss and Uncoupling of Receptors

It was shown convincingly that aging is accompanied by the progressive loss of a number of receptors.[18,19] The loss of important receptors as those mediating several hormone actions and the activity of the autonomous nervous system can be considered as important factors in the age-dependent loss of tissue- and cell homeostatic regulations.[20] We described a related process, the uncoupling of a receptor, the receptor recognising

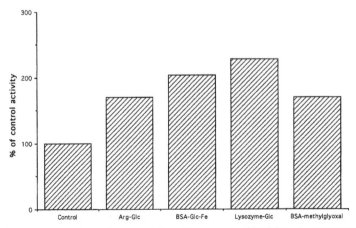

Fig. 5. Increase of elastase type endopeptidase activity of human skin fibroblasts in presence of AGE-products, in percent as compared to control (100%). AGE-products added: Arginin–glucose; bovine serum albumine–glucose-Fe; lysozyme–glucose and bovine serum albumin–methylglyoxal.

elastin peptide sequences.[21] The elastin-recognising subunit of this receptor has a second, galactose-recognising lectin site. Therefore, elastin sequences act as agonists and galactose-ending oligo- and polisaccharides act as antagonists. The message-transmission pathway was also described, both in human mononuclear cells and endothelial cells.[22–24] It appeared however that with age, the message transmission pathway became modified. Inhibitors of the first step of the transmission pathway from the receptor to the G-protein such as pertussis toxin could no more inhibit superoxide release from mononuclear cells taken from "old" individuals (>65 years) when elastin peptides were added (**Fig. 6**). This same inhibition was efficient in "young" cells (<45 years). There remained however the possibility to inhibit the upregulation of elastase-type endopeptidase release by fibroblasts in presence of elastin peptides by lactose or melibiose (**Fig. 6**). The affinity constant of the elastin receptor for elastin peptides did not change with age, it remained in the nanomolar range. Several other physiologically useful functions of the receptor vanished also with age, such as the dose-dependent inhibition of cholesterol biosynthesis from ^{14}C-acetate in monocytes[25] or the coupling of the receptor to iNOS in endothelial cells resulting in presence of elastin peptides in NO release and vasodilation.[26] The overall result of receptor uncoupling was therefore the loss of all physiologically useful effects of the elastin receptor with the maintenance of only the harmful effects such as upregulation of elastase-production and of free radical release. As elastin peptides are present in the blood and body fluids, the elastin receptor is constantly exposed to its agonists producing the above-mentioned harmful effects.

INHIBITION OF AGE-RELATED HARMFUL EFFECTS

Among the substances tested during our experiments, several classes of active principles proved efficient to inhibit one or several of the above-mentioned harmful effects. Inhibitors of the Maillard reaction were recently reviewed by Urios and colleagues.[27] The antagonists of the elastin receeptor such as melibiose were used with success (**Fig. 7**). During the last years, we mainly studied fucose- and rhamnose-rich oligo- and polysaccharides (FROP and RROP). They proved to be active in inhibiting most of the above-described harmful effects such as cytotoxicity of AGE-products (**Table 2**), the upregulation of elastase activity (**Fig. 6**) and stimulating cell proliferation and ECM-biosynthesis, in vitro as well as in vivo. They also were shown to counteract periorbital wrinkle formation.[28] Their mode of action was also studied. A fluorescent-labelled oligosaccharide, FROP-3, was shown to react with cell membrane localised receptors and also, surprisingly, to penetrate massively in the cell nucleus.[29–31]

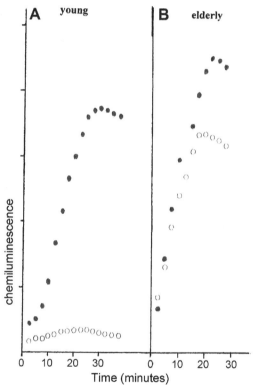

Fig. 6. Increase of superoxide release from human mononuclear cells in presence of κ-elastin, the agonist of the elastin receptor (●●●) and its inhibition by pertussis toxin which blocks the transmission pathway of the receptor at the level of the Gi-protein (ooo). This inhibition works only on cells from "young" individuals (<45 years) but does no more function with cells of "old" individuals (>65 years), sign of the uncoupling of the receptor (*Data from* Füllöp T, Daupiech N, Jacob MP, et al. Age related alterations in the signal transduction pathway of the elastin-laminin receptor. Pathol Biol 2001;49:339–48.).

DISCUSSION

Aging is a complex process, skin aging is no exception. No single process is adequate to describe and even less to "explain" it. Most well studied and reproducibly modelised processes involved in cell-tissue aging appear to belong to the epigenetic and post-translational mechanisms. This is the case for the decline of cell proliferation by exit from the mitotic pool, of the decline

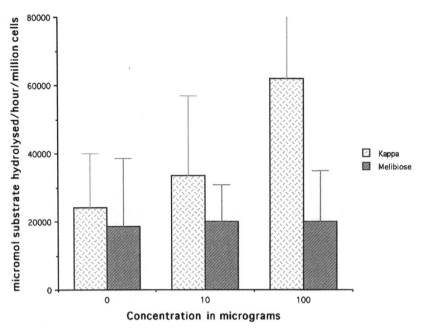

Fig. 7. Increase of elastase-type activity of human skin fibroblasts in presence of elastin peptides (κ-elastin) and its inhibition by an antagonist of the elastin-receptor, melibiose. Clear columns: kappa-elastin added at indicated concentration. Blue columns: kappa-elastin and melibiose added.

of ECM-biosynthesis and increasing matrix-degradation. The detailed study of the involved mechanisms revealed some interesting features of such processes clearly involved in age-dependent decline of cell-tissue function. This is the case for the production of harmful peptides during proteolytic degradation of finbronectine and of elastin, analysed in some detail above. The Maillard reaction is no exception, there is no life without sugar (glucose) but part of this essential nutrient is deviated from the (genetically "programmed") metabolic pathway to entertain harmful processes. These processes, AGE-production, is the result of a simple organic reaction, glycosylamine formation followed by more complex reactions, not forseen by the "genetic program". The conclusion proposed by Jacob[32] is unavoidable. Nature is tinkering instead of producing masterpieces.[32] As analysed in detail in a previous monography[33] the bio-logics of aging did not arise as a result of life-saving processes. On the contrary, most life-supporting molecular processes appear to produce harmful by-products. This is the case of oxydative phosphorylation in mitochondria, site of active release of free radicals and also of receptor production and

Table 2
Protection by RROP against the toxic effect of AGE-products. Percentage protection against cell death (Table 1)

Substance Added to AGE-lysozyme	% Protection and Significance
RROP-2, 10 µg/ml	0%[b]
RROP-3, 10 µg/ml	47.3[d]
Substance Added to AGE-BSA	% Protection and Significance
RROP-2, 10 µg/ml	42[a]
RROP-3, 10 µg/ml	50.4[c]

[a] $p<.05$.
[b] $p<.01$.
[c] $p<.005$.
[d] $p<.001$.

function as illustrated above. There is however a practically exploitable aspect of such post-translational mechanisms. They are much easier to understand and modelised in order to be inhibited or at least slowed down as would be the case for genetically "coded" mechanisms, as for instance the pathologies resulting from gene-modifications, for example progeria. In order to be successful, however, tentatives to slow down or to inhibit age-related harmful processes, the most important requisite is their complete understanding and modeling.

ACKNOWLEDGMENTS

The original experiments mentioned in the text were supported by CNRS, Inserm and Institute DERM, Paris. We thankfully acknowledge the generous hospitality of Prof. Gilles Renard, Head of the Department of Ophthalmology. A number of co-workers participated over the years in the here-described experiments, their names can be found in the references.

REFERENCES

1. Browner WS, Kahn AJ, Ziv E, et al. The genetics of human longevity. Am J Med 2004;117:851–60.
2. Robert L, Labat-Robert J. Aging of connective tissues, from genetic to epigenetic mechanisms. Biogerontology 2000;1:123–31.
3. Guarente L, Picard F. Calorie restriction – the SIR2 connection. Cell 2005;120:473–82.
4. Mobbs CV, Yen K, Hof PR, editors. Mechanisms of dietary restriction in aging and disease. Basel: Karger; 2007.
5. Branchet MC, Boisnic S, Francès C, et al. Skin thickness changes in normal aging skin. Gerontology 1990;36:28–35.
6. Labat-Robert J, Robert L. The effect of cell-matrix interactions and aging on the malignant process. In: Van de Woude, Klein G, editors. Adv Cancer Res 2007;98:221–59.
7. McClintock D, Ratner D, Lokuge M, et al. The mutant form of lamin A that causes Hutchinson-Gilford progeria is a biomarker of cellular aging in human skin. PloS ONE 2:e1269. doi:10.1371/Journal.pone.0001269.
8. Hornebeck W, Derouette JC, Roland J, et al. Corrélation entre âge, l'artériosclérose et l'activité élastolytique de la paroi aortique humain. C R Acad Sci 1976;292:2003–6.
9. Labat-Robert J, Fourtanier A, Boyer-Lafargue B, et al. Age-dependent increase of elastase-type protease activity in mouse skin. Effect of UV-irradiation. J Photochem Photobiol 2000;57:113–8.
10. Robert L, Molinari J, Ravelojaona V, et al. Age-and passage-dependent upregulation of fibroblast elastase-type endopeptidase activity. Role of advanced glycation endproducts, inhibition by fucose- and rhamnose-rich oligosaccharides. Arch Gerontol geriatr 2010;50:327–31.
11. Verzar F. The aging of collagen. Sci Am 1963;204:104–14.
12. Robert L. Fritz Verzar was born 120 years ago: his contribution to experimental gerontology through the collagen research as assessed after half a century. Arch Gerontol Geriatr 2006;43:13–43.
13. Baynes JW, Monnier VM, Ames JM, et al, editors. The Maillard reaction. Chemistry at the interface of nutrition, aging and disease. Ann New York Acad Sci 2005;1043.
14. Péterszegi G, Molinari J, Ravelojaona V, et al. Effect of advanced glycation end-products on cell proliferation and cell death. Pathol Biol 2006;54:396–404.
15. Vlassara H. Advanced glycation in health and disease. Role of modern environment. Ann N Y Acad Sci 2005;1043:452–60.
16. Labat-Robert J. Fibronectin in malignancy. Effect of aging. Semin Cancer Biol 2002;12:187–95.
17. Labat-Robert J. Cell-matrix interactions in aging: role of receptors and matricriptins. Ageing Res Rev 2004;3:233–47.
18. Roth GS. Changes in tissue responsiveness to hormones and neurotransmitters during aging. Exp Gerontol 1995;30:361–8.
19. Lakatta EG. Deficient neuroendocrine regulation of the cardiovascular system with advancing age in healthy humans. Circulation 1993;87:631–6.
20. Robert L. Mechanisms of aging of the extracellular matrix. Role of the elastin-laminin receptor. Novartis Price Lecture. Gerontology 1998;44:307–17.
21. Fülöp T, Daupiech N, Jacob MP, et al. Age related alterations in the signal transduction pathway of the elastin-laminin receptor. Pathol Biol 2001;49:339–48.
22. Varga Z, Jacob MP, Robert L, et al. Identification and signal transduction mechanism of elastine peptide receptor in human leukocytes. FEBS Lett 1989;258:5–8.
23. Faury G, Usson Y, Robert-Nicoud M, et al. Nuclear and cytoplasmic free calcium level changes induced by elastin peptides in human endothelial cells. Proc Natl Acad Sci U S A 1998;95:2967–72.
24. Faury G, Garbier S, Weiss AS, et al. Action of tropoelastin and synthetic elastin sequences on vascular tone and on free calcium level in human vascular endothelial cells. Circ Res 1998;82:328–36.
25. Varga Zs, Jacob MP, Robert L, et al. Age-dependent changes of kappa-elastin stimulated effector functions of human phagocytic cells: relevance for atherogenesis. Exp Gerontol 1997;32:653–62.
26. Faury G, Chabaud A, Ristori MT, et al. Effect of age on the vasodilatory action of elastin peptides. Mech Ageing Dev 1997;95:31–42.

27. Urios P, Grigorova-Borsos AM, Peyroux J, et al. Inhibition de la glycation avancée par les flavonoïdes. Implication nutritionnelle dans la prévention des complications du diabète ? J Soc Biol 2007;201:189–98.

28. Robert C, Robert AM, Robert L. Effect of a preparation containing a fucose-rich polysaccharide on periorbital wrinkles of human voluntaries. Skin Res Technol 2004;10:16.

29. Péterszegi G, Fodil-Bourahla I, Robert AM, et al. Pharmacological properties of fucose Applications in age-related modifications of connective tissues. Biomed Pharmacother 2003;57:240–5.

30. Péterszegi G, Isnard N, Robert AM, et al. Studies on skin aging. Preparation and properties of fucose-rich oligo- and polysaccharides. Effect on fibroblast

proliferation and survival. Biomed Pharmacother 2003;57:187–94.

31. Andrès E, Molinari J, Péterszegi G, et al. Pharmacological properties of rhamnose-rich poloysaccharides, potential interest in age-dependent alterations of connective tissues. Pathol Biol 2006;54:420–5.

32. Jacob F. Evolution and tinkering. Science 1977;196. 1161.

33. Robert L, Miquel PA. Bio-logiques du vieillissement. Éditions KIME; 2004.

34. Ravelojaona V, Robert AM, Robert L. Expression of senescence-associated β-galactosidase by human skin fibroblasts. Effect of advanced glycation end-products and fucose- or rhamnose-rich polysaccharides. Arch Gerontol Geriatr 2008. DOI:10.1016/ j.archger.2007.12.004.

Stiffening of Human Skin Fibroblasts with Age

Christian Schulze[a,b,*], Franziska Wetzel[a],
Thomas Kueper[b], Anke Malsen[b], Gesa Muhr[b],
Soeren Jaspers[b], Thomas Blatt[b], Klaus-Peter Wittern[b],
Horst Wenck[b], Josef A. Käs[a]

KEYWORDS

- Aging skin • Human dermal fibroblasts (HDF)
- Skin fibroblasts • Cellular function • Cellular senescence
- Viscoelasticity

INTRODUCTION

Aging is the result of a complex interaction of biological, physical, and biochemical processes that cause changes and damage to molecules, cellular function, and organs. To date, several studies have examined age-related alterations in cell division, biosynthesis,[1–3] and cell migration,[4] but there is little information about the relationship between aging and the mechanical properties of cells. Previous studies have shown that biomechanical properties are important for cell functions that are regulated by mechanical forces.[5,6] Individual cells are able to sense mechanical signals and transduce them into a biochemical response. When the synthesis activity of cells is compared in stressed versus relaxed collagen gels, as well as for cells growing in collagen gels versus plastic dishes,[7–10] a link is observed between the collagen production of fibroblasts and the mechanical forces acting on the cells. This is not surprising, since active and passive cellular biomechanics based on the stability provided by the cytoskeleton impacts many essential cellular functions. In addition to the role of the cytoskeleton in cellular motility and division,[11,12] it has been shown that a functionally intact cytoskeleton is crucial to build up contraction forces in a three-dimensional collagen lattice.[13,14] These cell functions are essential for the homeostasis of the extracellular matrix (ECM).

Considering the importance of cellular biomechanics for correct physiological functioning, we analyzed the mechanical behavior of dermal fibroblasts isolated from human donors of different ages. Changes in mechanical properties of the skin are generally referred to extracellular aspects such as alterations in polymerization and cross-linking of collagen and elastin.[15] In this context, age-related changes have been observed for protein synthesis and production of ECM components.[1,16,17] Further, atomic force microscopy studies indicate that individual epithelial cells show a considerable increase in stiffness in vitro at higher passage numbers.[18,19] Even though comparisons of cells of early and late passage have yielded important insights into the aging process in vitro, such models cannot substitute for studies of cells isolated from aged human donors (aged in vivo). Thus far, no study has compared the viscoelastic properties of dermal fibroblasts from young and advanced-age donors. To address this issue, the optical stretcher technique was applied to examine the deformability of fibroblasts isolated from 14 human donors.

The microfluidic optical stretcher is an optical trap that allows trapping and controlled deformation of

This article originally published in *Biophysical Journal 99(8), 2010*.
[a] Division of Soft Matter Physics, Department of Physics, University of Leipzig, Leipzig, Germany
[b] R&D, Beiersdorf, Hamburg, Germany
* Corresponding author.
E-mail address: chr-s@gmx.de

Clin Plastic Surg 39 (2012) 9–20
doi:10.1016/j.cps.2011.09.008

suspended cells using two counterpropagating laser beams.[20] Cellular extension is caused by a momentum transfer acting on the cell surface. The global stress applied by the optical stretcher permits the measurement of whole-cell elasticity that characterizes the integral effects of molecular changes on the cytoskeleton. The use of optical deformability as a sensitive cell marker has already been demonstrated for characterization of individual cancer cell lines,[21] as well as for cancer diagnosis by mechanical phenotyping of oral keratinocytes.[22] We suggest that optical deformability can also serve as a sensitive biomarker of aging on the level of individual dermal cells. To date, cellular senescence as a measure of aging has been characterized by molecular markers based on an altered pattern of gene and protein expression. Typical known biomarkers are senescence-associated β-galactosidase,[23] telomere dysfunction,[24,25] expression of activated p53 and p16,[25,26] and nuclear accumulation of globular actin.[27]

Since viscoelastic properties are determined by the cytoskeletal polymers, and actin is supposed to be a key element,[28,29] we further quantified the amount of polymerized actin using FACS measurements. In addition, possible age-related changes in vimentin and microtubule content were analyzed. In vivo, there are many cells able to perform mechanical work, for example, muscle cells or cells of connective tissues that are connected to the proteins of the ECM. Three-dimensional collagen lattices seeded with fibroblasts have been used to analyze the effect of actin or microtubule disruption on the mechanical activity of cells.[13,14] The mechanical properties of cells and the state of the cytoskeleton affect the interaction between fibroblasts and the ECM,[30–32] so mechanical changes may reveal new aspects of the age-related degradation of the elastic properties of the dermis. Rheological measurements were used to characterize fibroblast-populated collagen gels as dermis equivalents. These experiments determine the influence of changes in the mechanical properties of cells and the cytoskeleton on the organization and mechanical behavior of the collagen matrix.

MATERIALS AND METHODS
Cell Culture

Biopsies were isolated from plastic surgery procedures. We adhered to the recommendations of the current version of the Declaration of Helsinki as applied to a non-drug study. All donors provided written, informed consent. Human dermal fibroblasts (HDFs) were isolated by outgrowth from skin biopsy samples obtained from healthy female donors of different ages (20–80 years). Primary cells were enzymatically prepared using a dispase digestion technique. Square-cut biopsy pieces were washed, rinsed, and incubated in dispase (Boehringer Mannheim, Mannheim, Germany) for 2 h at 37°C and 7% CO_2. The dermis and epidermis were then separated and the dermal fraction was cultured in six-well plates containing Dulbecco's modified Eagle's medium (Life Technologies, Eggenstein, Germany) supplemented with 10% fetal calf serum (Life Technologies) and penicillin/streptomycin (50 μg/ml, Life Technologies). Confluent fibroblasts were seeded into appropriate flasks. For the experiments, cells were used at passage 3 grown to 90% confluency. Generally, the two age groups were defined as young donors <42 years and old donors >60 years. Due to limited biopsy material, donor ages can vary between different experiments.

Refractive Index Measurements

The refractive indices of fibroblast populations from different-aged donors were measured using a phase-matching technique.[33–35] Cells are suspended in bovine serum albumin (BSA) phosphate-buffered saline solutions with different concentrations of BSA. Since the refractive index of the solution depends on the protein concentration, the refractive index of the surrounding medium is varied.

The exact refractive index of each solution is measured using an Abbe-refractometer (AR4, Krüss Optronics, Hamburg, Germany) and the appearance of the cells in a phase-contrast microscope is analyzed. Cells with an index of refraction lower than the surrounding medium are brighter than the background, and cells with a higher refractive index appear dark (Fig. S8 A in the Supporting Material). Assuming a normal distribution for the refractive indices of the cells, the percentage of cells that appear brighter than the background can be fitted by an error function (Fig. S8 B):

$$f(n) = \frac{1}{\sigma \times \sqrt{2\pi}} \times \int_{-\infty}^{n} e^{\frac{(x-\mu)^2}{2\sigma^2}} dx. \tag{1}$$

Here, σ is the standard deviation of the distribution and μ is the mean value of the refractive index, which corresponds to the inflection point of the error function. Both parameters are determined by the fit of the data.

Optical Stretcher

The optical stretcher is an optical trap consisting of two coaxially aligned, counterpropagating divergent laser beams that apply optical forces to the surfaces of suspended cells.[20,21] Increasing the laser power will deform the whole cell along the laser-beam axis. The stretching is caused by transfer of momentum to the cell membrane pointing away from the medium of higher refractive index.[21,36] Stress magnitude and distribution can be calculated by a ray optics approach. A schematic of a resulting stress profile acting on the cell surface is shown in **Fig. 1**A.

The setup consists of an ytterbium-doped fiber laser operating at a wavelength of 1064 nm (YLM-10-1064, IPG Photonics, Burbach, Germany) with a maximum output power of 10 W. The optical fiber was spliced to a 1 × 2 coupler, splitting the light in a 50:50 ratio. Cells were positioned between the two laser beams by a microfluidic delivery system[37] For this, a glass capillary tube (VitroCom, Mountain Lakes, NJ) was situated between the two fiber ends (**Fig. 1**B). The optical fibers (PureMode HI 1060, Corning, Wiesbaden, Germany) were placed at a distance of ~120 μm from the capillary wall. The whole microfluidic system was mounted on an inverted phase-contrast microscope (DMIL, Leica, Solms, Germany)

and deformations of the cells were recorded at a rate of 30 frames/s using a CCD camera (A202k, Basler, Ahrensburg, Germany). The images obtained were analyzed automatically by a LabView routine that determines the cell boundaries (**Fig. 1**A) and calculates the strain of the cells along the laser-beam axis.[20,21] The laser power used was P = 0.2 W/fiber for trapping the cells and P = 1.2 W/fiber for the stretching. The resulting extension behavior was analyzed, and viscoelastic properties of the cells were calculated as described in Wottawah et al.[38] In the three-parameter model used, optical deformability, which corresponds to the compliance of the cells, is described by

$$\gamma(t) = \sigma \left(\frac{b_1}{a_1} - \frac{a_2}{a_1^2} \right) \left(1 - e^{-\frac{a_1}{a_2}t} \right) + \frac{\sigma}{a_1}t \qquad (2)$$

when the stress is applied ($0 < t < t_1$) and by

$$\gamma(t) = \sigma \left(\frac{b_1}{a_1} - \frac{a_2}{a_1^2} \right) \left(1 - e^{-\frac{a_1}{a_2}t_1} \right) e^{-\frac{a_1}{a_2}(t-t_1)} + \frac{\sigma}{a_1}t$$

$$(3)$$

when the laser is off again ($t > t_1$). Here, σ represents the applied stress and a_1, a_2, and b_1 are parameters derived from the viscoelastic constitutive equation. Further information about calculation of the stress, σ, can be found in Guck et al.[20] and Wottawah et al.[38] The constants can be obtained by fitting the data to allow the calculation of rheological parameters like the plateau Young's modulus, E_p, which is a measure of the overall elastic behavior of cells:

$$E_p = \lim_{\omega \to \infty} E'(\omega) = \frac{a_1 b_1 - a_2}{b_1^2}. \qquad (4)$$

FACS Analysis

After incubation of fibroblasts to a confluence level of 90%, cells were trypsinized, centrifuged at 10,000 rpm, and washed twice with PBS. Cells were then resuspended in 3% paraformaldehyde and incubated for 30 min at room temperature. After two additional washing steps, the cells were permeabilized with 0.5% Triton-X100 (Sigma, St. Louis, MO) in PBS. Cells were then washed, blocked for 30 min with 3% BSA, and washed again. For actin staining, Alexa-488-labeled Dnase I and Alexa-647-labeled phalloidin (Invitrogen, Paisley, United Kingdom) were added at concentrations of 161.0 μM and 6.6 μM, respectively. Cells were incubated for 20 min at room temperature. After two washing steps with PBS, the fluorescence was measured using

A

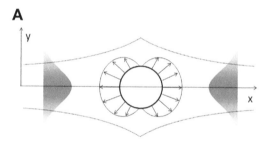

B

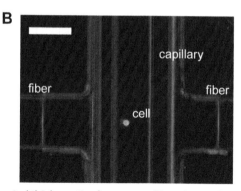

Fig. 1. (A) Schematic of a stress profile acting on the cell surface due to momentum transfer caused by two divergent laser beams with Gaussian intensity profile. The peak stress along the laser beam axis depends on the laser power and refractive indices of the cell and the surrounding medium. (B) Optical stretcher setup. Two opposing optical fibers are aligned perpendicular to a glass capillary holding a suspended cell. Scale bar, 50 μm (*From* Lincoln B, Wottawah F, Guck J. High-throughput rheological measurements with an optical stretcher. Methods Cell Biol 2007;83:397–423; with permission.).

a FACSCanto flow cytometer (BD Biosciences, San Jose, CA) and analyzed by the software BD FACSDiva 4.0.

Concerning microtubule staining, the cells were incubated for 30 min with Oregon Green 488 conjugated paclitaxel (Invitrogen) at a concentration of 1.0 μM. Vimentin was detected using an antibody (sc-32322, dilution 1:200) purchased from Santa Cruz Biotechnology (Santa Cruz, CA).

Tissue Rheology

For preparation of dermis equivalents, 100 mg Type I collagen (Sigma, St. Louis, MO) was dissolved at 4°C in 33.3 ml of 0.1% sterile acetic acid (c = 3 mg/ml). The used fibroblast populated gels consist of 80% collagen solution, 10% 10× Hanks' buffer salt solution (Biochrom, Berlin, Germany), and 10% fetal calf serum containing 3×10^6 suspended cells/ml. The final solution contained 2.4 mg/ml collagen and 3×10^5 fibroblasts/ml. NaOH (1 M) was added dropwise to neutralize the solution, whereof 2.5 ml was applied to six-well plates (Greiner, Germany) and incubated at 37°C and 7% CO_2 for 1 h. The gels were covered with 2 ml medium (DMEM, 1% penicillin/streptomycin, 1% glutamax, and 10% FCS) and incubated for another 23 h at 37°C and 7% CO_2. To study the specific effect of cytoskeletal stiffening, collagen gels were treated for 48 h with 0.5 μM jasplakinolide in DMEM. Jasplakinolide is described as promoting actin polymerization and stabilizes actin filaments, leading to increased cellular stiffness.[38,39] A possible connection between actin stabilization and cellular aging has already been hypothesized by Gourlay et al.[41] who measured an increased reactive oxygen species production in connection with decreased actin turnover induced by jasplakinolide. Although the effect of jasplakinolide treatment is controversial in literature,[42] optical stretcher experiments confirmed a higher cell stiffness after drug treatment (Fig. S10).

Viscoelastic properties of the gels were measured by a shear rheometer (AR2000ex, TA Instruments, New Castle, DE) using a plate-plate geometry (diameter, 2 cm). The AR2000ex offers different modes of oscillatory experiments to determine the complex shear modulus, $G^* = G' + iG''$, which depends on shear frequency, stress, and strain. Fibroblast-populated collagen gels were characterized by measurement of the elastic storage modulus, G', and the viscous loss modulus, G'', in the linear viscoelastic regime ($\gamma = 2\%$ and $\omega = 5$ rad/s). At higher deformation, plastic effects were observed in the form of decreasing storage moduli.

RESULTS

The microfluidic optical stretcher was used to determine the viscoelastic properties, i.e., stiffness, of dermal fibroblasts as a function of donor age. The optical stretcher uses two opposing divergent laser beams to trap and stretch a cell along the laser-beam axis with increasing laser power.[20] To compare the optical deformability of cells, it has to be considered that the stretching forces acting on the cell surface crucially depend on the relative refractive index of the cell population and the surrounding medium. That means a cell with a higher refractive index gets more stretched. We determined the refractive indices of fibroblast populations from six different donors using a phase-matching technique described by Barer and Joseph.[33–35] Briefly summarized, the percentage of bright and dark cells compared to the surrounding medium is evaluated by varying optical density of the medium. Fitting an error function to the data provides the distribution of refractive indices of the cells. The differences in optical properties for the tested cell populations were within statistical error, with a mean refractive index of 1.368 (Supporting Material). Since fibroblasts isolated from different donors cannot be distinguished based on their refractive index, differences in optical deformability can be attributed solely to the mechanical properties of the cells.

To elucidate the relationship between aging and the viscoelastic properties of cells, basic rheologic-step stress experiments were performed with the optical stretcher. Suspended fibroblasts were trapped at a laser power of 200 mW and deformed for 2 s at a constant power of 1.2 W/fiber resulting in a peak stress of ∼1.8 Pa along the laser-beam axis. During the stretch, the relative radial extension, i.e., the strain, $\gamma(t)$, is monitored. After the laser was switched back to trapping power ($t>3$ s), the relaxation behavior was also observed. **Fig. 2**A shows the typical viscoelastic extension behavior of two fibroblast populations from different-aged donors. The mean deformability of a cell population, together with the standard error of the mean as a function of time, was determined for every frame recorded. Cells of a 73-year-old donor showed a significantly higher stiffness, leading to decreased deformation compared to those of the 27-year-old donor. Sample sizes in this experiment were $n_{young} = 30$ cells and $n_{old} = 24$ cells. Assuming a normal distribution, histograms of the deformability at maximum strain were fitted as illustrated in **Fig. 2**B. Student's t-test demonstrates that the two samples belong to different populations with a probability of 99%.

A

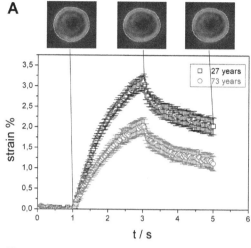

B

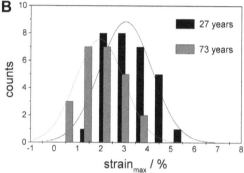

Fig. 2. (*A*) Time-dependent deformation behavior of two fibroblast populations. Cells are stretched for 2 s at a laser power of 1.2 W/fiber in a step-stress experiment and the viscoelastic extension is measured. Error bars show the standard error of the mean. Fibroblasts of an old donor (73 years) show lower deformability resulting in a maximum strain $\gamma_{max} = 2.04\% \pm 0.19\%$ along the laser beam axis compared to cells of a young donor (27 years; maximum strain, $\gamma_{max} = 3.12\% \pm 0.18\%$). (*B*) Histograms of the maximum strain. A Student's *t*-test (*P*<.01) indicates that the separation into two populations based on maximum deformability is statistically significant.

Since maximum deformation does not reflect the overall viscoelastic behavior of the cells and uses only a small part of the information provided by the stress-deformation experiments, we also calculated rheological parameters, namely the time- and frequency-dependent elastic moduli. As described in Wottawah et al.[38] these parameters can be derived from optical deformability, which is in general a function of time and corresponds to the compliance of the cells (see Supporting Material). The overall viscoelastic behavior can be characterized by the modulus functions E(t), the time-dependent Young's modulus, and

$E^*(\omega) = E'(\omega) + E''(\omega)$, the frequency-dependent complex Young's modulus.

$E'(\omega)$ is a measure of the elastic energy stored in the sample during a periodic deformation and is also called the storage modulus. $E''(\omega)$ is the loss modulus, which represents the viscous dissipation of energy. E(t) describes the stress relaxation behavior of the cells. Typical graphs of these rheological properties are given in **Fig. 3**, A and B, and allow the calculation of characteristic material constants such as the elastic plateau modulus, E_p (**Fig. 3**A), for short times and high frequencies. To compare the age-dependent elastic behavior of fibroblast populations of different donors, we determined the plateau modulus and found a significant increase in stiffness at higher ages (**Fig. 3**, C and D). Examining differences between the two age groups, 27–42 years and 61–80 years, the mean plateau modulus was found to range from 143.6 ± 38.3 Pa for the young cell populations to 235.2 ± 29.9 Pa in the elderly group, which is a considerable shift of ∼60% (*P* = 0.005, Mann-Whitney U-Test). To put this into perspective, the malignant transformation of a fibroblast causes a 30% higher compliance.[38] This drastic effect is somewhat surprising and could not be anticipated from previous literature.

Since the state of actin polymerization and the organization of actin filaments is widely believed to be related to the mechanical properties of cells,[28,29] the intracellular monomer (G-) and filamentous (F-) actin content was measured by FACS analysis. We compared the degree of polymerized actin for cells of young and old donors by dual fluorescence labeling using Alexa-647 phalloidin and Alexa-488 DNase I. Since the labeling of F-actin and G-actin with phalloidin and DNase I, respectively, is known to be specific and the staining patterns are thought to be spatially separate and distinct,[43] this method allowed us to measure the relative amounts of G- and F-actin in the same cell simultaneously. As can be seen by confocal microscopy (**Fig. 4**A), the F-actin polymer network forms a dense cortical layer underneath the plasma membrane even when the cells are in suspension. G-actin is distributed throughout the cytoplasm. Some cells also show a nuclear accumulation of G-actin, but the possible correlation with donor age described by Kwak et al.[27] was not observed. **Fig. 4**, B and C, shows typical fluorescence intensity distributions, obtained by FACS, for the fibroblast populations of a young and an old donor. An increase in the F-actin level is clearly visible for the older donor. To quantify the state of actin polymerization, we determined the G-actin/F-actin signal ratio for a total of 12 donors. The statistical results are given in **Fig. 4**,

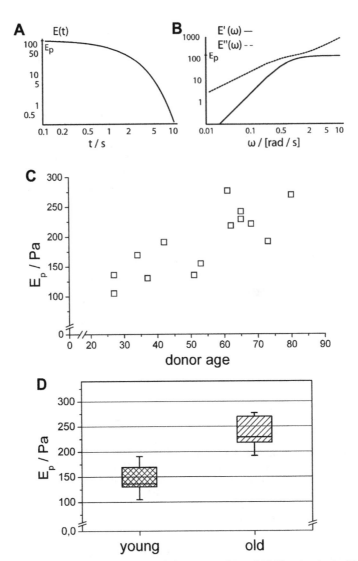

Fig. 3. The relation between fibroblast elasticity and donor age. (*A* and *B*) The rheological behavior of cells can be characterized by time- (*A*) and frequency-dependent (*B*) modulus functions derived from the temporal development of strain (**Fig. 2**A).[21] (*C*) As a measure of the elastic strength of the cells, we calculated the plateau Young's modulus, E_p, for all optical stretcher experiments. We identified an age-related increase in cell stiffness. (*D*) The plateau modulus for the donor age group 27–42 years is significantly shifted to higher values in the age group 61–80 years, with a confidence level of >99% (Mann-Whitney U-test).

D–F. Comparison of the two age groups, 20–27 years (n = 6) and 61–72 years (n = 6), shows that the balance between F- and G-actin is altered in favor of F-actin by ~31% (*P* = 0.007, Mann-Whitney U-test). This shift is basically due to an increased F-actin level. Due to its location just beneath the plasma membrane and its high mechanical strength, the actin cortex is thought to dominate the viscoelastic response of the cells to small deformations. The result confirms the hypothesis that the changes in mechanical properties observed are linked to an altered degree of actin polymerization in cells of old individuals.

To elucidate possible age-related changes of expression of the other cytoskeletal components (microtubules and vimentin), we compared the corresponding intracellular content of fibroblasts isolated from young (20–35 years) and old (60–76 years) donors. After fixation and permeabilization of suspended cells, microtubules and vimentin were stained and fluorescence intensities were quantified by FACS. For both cytoskeletal polymers, a statistically insignificant decrease of the FACS signals was observed at higher donor ages (**Fig. 5**). A possible correlation between increased cell stiffness and higher microtubule and vimentin content could

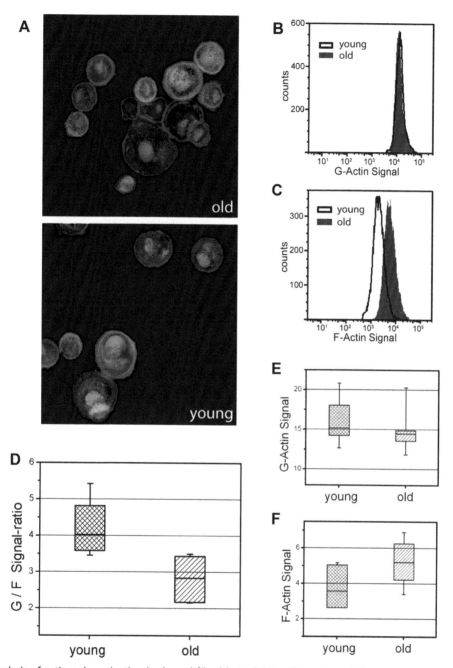

Fig. 4. Analysis of actin polymerization in dermal fibroblasts. (*A*) For illustration of the actin staining, representative fluorescence confocal images of the F-actin cortex (*red*) and G-actin monomers (*green*) in suspended cells obtained from a young and an old donor are shown. Actin filaments form a homogeneous layer just beneath the plasma membrane. The fluorescence signals were quantified by FACS measurements to determine the state of actin polymerization. (*B* and *C*) Typical intensity distributions for the cells of an old and a young donor. Analyzing the G-/F-actin signal ratio in connection with donor age, we found a statistically significant shift to the polymerized state ($P = 0.007$, Mann-Whitney U-test) (*D*). Separate examination of G- and F-actin signals shows that this alteration results primarily from an increased F-actin fraction in fibroblasts of old donors (*E* and *F*).

not be confirmed. Nevertheless, we cannot rule out the possibility that some other events, such as changes in filament organization and cross-linking, contribute to the increased cell stiffness.

The cytoskeleton is the source of mechanical activity of fibroblasts, which is thought to participate in the structural constitution of the dermis and its physiological tension. The impact of

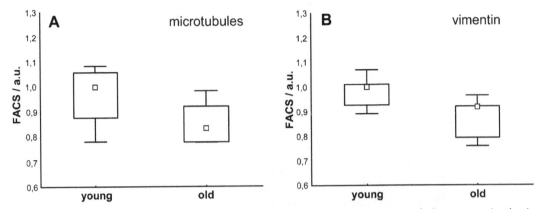

Fig. 5. (*A*) Analysis of age-related changes of the microtubule cytoskeleton. Microtubules were stained using paclitaxel (Oregon Green 488 Taxol) and signals were quantified by FACS measurement. This comparison of cells obtained from young and old donors does not show statistically significant differences ($P = 0.13$, Mann-Whitney U-test) but does show a slight decrease in signal intensity. (*B*) Fluorescence signals of vimentin also show a nonsignificant decrease at higher donor age ($P = 0.10$).

changing the cytoskeleton and cell elasticity on the constitution of the extracellular matrix was analyzed by tissue rheology. Dermal fibroblasts from different-aged donors or specifically modified actin cytoskeleton were seeded out in collagen gels to study the mechanical interaction between the cells and the ECM. Dermis equivalents were prepared as described in Materials and Methods and a shear rheometer was used to apply an oscillatory shear stress and measure the mechanical properties of the sample expressed by the complex shear modulus, $G^* = G' + iG''$. As a measure of the elastic response of fibroblast-populated collagen gels, the storage modulus, G', was determined at a shear rate of $\omega = 5$ rad/s and a maximum strain of $\gamma = 2\%$. In the linear-viscoelastic regime, the storage modulus is independent of strain. At higher deformations (>4%), shear modulus values decline (data not shown), indicating measurement-generated irreversible plastic damage of the collagen gel, which should be avoided. The loss modulus, G'', reflects the viscous material properties associated with the energy loss in the sample. The results for six individual experiments are given in **Fig. 6**. In each experiment, cells of a young and an old donor were used, and the storage and loss moduli were measured for three to four gels. Fibroblast-populated collagen gels exhibit elastic rather than viscous behavior, observed as significantly higher values of G' compared to G''. Gels containing cells of old donors have less mechanical strength, shown by lower values of G' and G''. In summary, the median of the storage modulus, G', decreases by ~11.2% and that of the loss modulus, G'', by ~11.7%. Since a direct comparison between individual experiments is not feasible because there is

a new preparation of collagen solution in each case, a Wilcoxon test for paired samples was used for statistical analysis. Age-related differences in the mechanical properties of the gels are significant ($P = 0.046$ for G' and 0.028 for G''). This result has not been described previously in the literature, to our knowledge, and it shows that reorganization of the collagen matrix according to the cells brought into the gel directly influences its mechanical properties.

In addition to analyzing differences in gel properties depending on donor age, the effect of a specific modulation of the actin cytoskeleton of cells was measured. Treatment with jasplakinolide stabilizes actin filaments and was used to model the age-related increase in cell stiffness. Collagen gels were incubated for 24 h in cell culture medium. After that, 0.5 µM jasplakinolide was added, followed by another 48 h of incubation. Six individual experiments with cells of different-aged donors show that jasplakinolide treatment not only increases cell stiffness[40] but also influences the viscoelastic properties of the collagen matrix (**Fig. 7**). In each experiment, rheological behavior was compared between three treated and three control gels (shear frequency, $\omega = 5$ rad/s; shear deformation, $\gamma = 2\%$). The median of the storage modulus, G', shows an average decrease of ~12.8% in the case of jasplakinolide treatment. The loss modulus, G'', decreases by ~15.0%. A Wilcoxon test confirms that the observed changes in mechanical properties are statistically significant ($P = 0.028$ for G' and 0.028 for G''). The increased stiffness of the actin cytoskeleton caused by jasplakinolide results in altered rheological behavior of the collagen matrix, which reveals a connection between cell mechanics and the elasticity of dermal tissues. Decreased

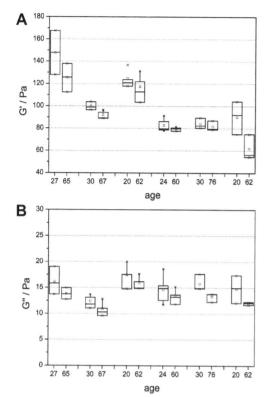

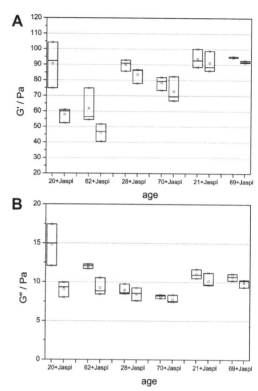

Fig. 6. Rheological properties of fibroblast-populated collagen gels depending on donor age. (*A*) In six individual experiments, three to four gels with cells of a young and an old donor were analyzed using a shear frequency of 5 rad/s and a strain of 2%. A significant decrease of G′ was observed (*P* = 0.046, Wilcoxon test). (*B*) The loss modulus, G″, shows a statistically significant decrease with age (*P* = 0.028, Wilcoxon test). These measurements demonstrate that collagen gels reorganized by aged fibroblasts exhibit less mechanical strength compared to those reorganized by cells of younger individuals.

Fig. 7. Storage (*A*) and loss (*B*) moduli of fibroblast-populated collagen gels measured at a shear frequency of 5 rad/s and a strain of 2%. In each of six individual experiments, six gels with cells of the same donor were analyzed, whereas three gels were treated for 48 h with 0.5 μM jasplakinolide. The increased cytoskeletal stiffness resulted in statistically significant decreases in the value of G′ and G″ (*P* = 0.028 for G′ and 0.028 for G″, Wilcoxon test), which clarifies that a specific modulation of the actin cytoskeleton has a direct effect on the mechanical behavior of the collagen matrix.

cell viability due to jasplakinolide treatment was excluded by an MTT vitality test.

DISCUSSION

Our results show that cellular stiffness is significantly increased in dermal fibroblasts during aging in vivo. The mechanical properties were assessed by measurements of the optical deformability of suspended cells with the optical stretcher. The ability to actually measure significant differences among cells of individual donors depending on age shows how sensitive optical deformability is to changes in structural composition of cells and indicates its potential as a biomarker of aging on the cellular level.

The experiments performed are based on probing the global rheological properties of cells in suspension. Although this may be considered nonphysiological because of the lack of contact with the extracellular matrix, nevertheless, the symmetric shell-like structural design and continuous distribution of stress over the cell surface allow measurement of whole-cell elasticity, i.e., the integrated state of the cytoskeleton, at a high throughput. In addition, the adherence of cells to a hard substrate like culture dishes or microscope slides does not reflect the situation of cells in vivo either, and measuring the mechanical properties of adhered cells using methods like atomic force microscopy (AFM) can introduce artifacts due to mechanical contact and an inhomogeneous cell morphology. By contrast, the optical stretcher allows for capturing effects of molecular changes that are reflected in the entire state of the cytoskeleton. Thus, the measurements with the optical stretcher may not directly reflect the viscoelastic properties of cells as found in a tissue matrix. However, they are a sensitive measure of the state of the cytoskeleton after isolation, which in consequence is responsible for a cell's mechanical stability.

The cytoskeleton is composed of actin, microtubules, and intermediate filaments and is regulated by a set of accessory proteins that can polymerize, cap, sever, cross-link, and bundle the polymers. By adding specific cytoskeleton-disrupting drugs and measuring the effect on cell elasticity, Rotsch et al.[29] demonstrated that the actin cytoskeleton plays a dominant role in a cell's mechanical stability. This is consistent with results from polymer physics showing that a network formed by the semiflexible actin filaments exhibits a higher resistance to an applied shear stress than microtubule and intermediate filament networks.[28] We found that depolymerization of F-actin using cytochalasin D leads to a significant increase in optical deformability up to 60% depending on donor age (Supporting Material). The crucial importance of the actin network for the mechanical properties of cells is also confirmed by our results showing that the degree of actin polymerization in fibroblasts of older individuals is shifted toward the filamentous form. This suggests that age-associated loss of cell flexibility is rooted in an altered polymerization of the actin cytoskeleton.

These are important findings, since the cytoskeleton and the mechanical properties of cells are essential for the organization of the collagen matrix, tissue development, and wound healing.[15,44] The actin cytoskeleton is responsible for cell contraction, which could be shown by the inhibition of contraction force generation for cytochalasin-D-treated fibroblasts.[13] Even concentrations of the F-actin disrupting drug as low as 2 nM lead to a significant alteration of the mechanical properties of a fibroblast-populated collagen matrix.[45] Further, Reed et al.[4] have shown that the age-related impairment in cell motility, which is a possible reason for delayed wound repair in dermal tissues, is accompanied by changes in cytoskeletal organization. Rao and Cohen already proposed that alterations in the actin cytoskeletal function may be an important aspect of generalized decrease in cellular function associated with aging.[46]

The changes found in the mechanical state and cytoskeletal organization of dermal fibroblasts reveal a new aspect of aging skin that could either directly or indirectly influence the viscoelastic behavior of the dermis. The age-associated impaired flexibility of the skin is generally attributed to a reduced density and modified architectural organization of collagen fibers,[15,47] an alteration of the elastic fiber network, and a reduction of the amount of proteoglycans.[48] The increased cell stiffness and higher actin polymerization could have a direct impact on cellular contraction capacity, as well as the organization and mechanical properties of the collagen matrix, since the actin cytoskeleton is an essential component of the interaction between fibroblasts and the ECM.[31] Here, it was shown, for the first time we know of, that increased cell stiffness affects the mechanical activity of dermal fibroblasts within the collagen matrix, resulting in lower shear-modulus values as the rheological analysis of fibroblast-populated collagen gels has shown. As a model of cytoskeletal aging, the reorganization of the ECM was inhibited by jasplakinolide treatment, which specifically stabilizes actin filaments.[39] This indicates a direct effect on skin structure and the mechanical properties of the dermis. The fact that collagen gels show an opposite trend compared to dermal cells, i.e., a decreased stiffness, seems nonintuitive and could be linked to a reduced contraction capacity of stiff fibroblasts (data not shown), leading to an altered structural organization and tension within the collagen matrix.

Besides this direct effect on the organization of the ECM, changes of the actin cytoskeleton could contribute to the altered gene expression in aged fibroblasts, leading to a reduced synthesis of ECM proteins. In recent years, it has become increasingly evident that the cytoskeleton and its mechanical state are key elements for mechanosensitivity and mechanotransduction,[6,49] which play an essential role in cellular regulation of differentiation, proliferation,[50] and gene expression.[8] Lambert et al.[7] demonstrated that synthesis of collagen and other extracellular matrix proteins is regulated by mechanical forces when comparing expression patterns of skin fibroblasts in stressed and relaxed collagen gels. Future work could clarify how age-related changes in the mechanical properties of cells, as observed in this study, influence the expression of ECM proteins.

Other cell functions, like motility and proliferation, could be affected by cytoskeletal changes. We assume a possible link between age-related changes in cell proliferation and the observed higher cell stiffness in connection with changes in actin organization. It has been shown that high proliferative cancer cells show a reduced degree of actin polymerization and mechanical strength.[21] Aging, on the other hand, leads to a high degree of actin polymerization, as we have shown, and decreased growth rate, as well as the replicative lifespan of a fibroblast culture.[51] A possible link of impaired motility and proliferation to age-related diseases could be especially relevant in the context of wound healing.

To date, molecular markers based on an altered pattern of gene and protein expression have been used to characterize cellular senescence as a measure of aging. The objective of a biomarker of aging is to reflect physiological function and help to monitor treatment response. Since the mechanical properties of cells are linked to their cytoskeletal structure, which in turn is governed by cellular function, optical deformability as measured with the optical stretcher appears to be a sensitive marker for cellular aging. Guck et al.[21] have already demonstrated the potential of optical deformability as a diagnostic marker for cancerous cells. We suggest that measurement of the global deformation behavior of individual cells also offers a novel, to our knowledge, cytological alternative to the genomic and proteomic techniques characterizing cellular senescence.

SUPPORTING MATERIAL

Equations and figures are available at http://www.biophysj.org/biophysj/supplemental/S0006-3495(10)00995-1.

This study was funded by the Federal Ministry of Education and Research (BMBF).

REFERENCES

1. Takeda K, Gosiewska A, Peterkofsky B. Similar, but not identical, modulation of expression of extracellular matrix components during in vitro and in vivo aging of human skin fibroblasts. J Cell Physiol 1992;153:450–9.

2. Cristofalo VJ, Allen RG, Beck JC, et al. Relationship between donor age and the replicative lifespan of human cells in culture: a reevaluation. Proc Natl Acad Sci USA 1998;95:10614–9.

3. Rattan SI. Theories of biological aging: genes, proteins, and free radicals. Free Radic Res 2006; 40:1230–8.

4. Reed MJ, Ferara NS, Vernon RB. Impaired migration, integrin function, and actin cytoskeletal organization in dermal fibroblasts from a subset of aged human donors. Mech Ageing Dev 2001;122:1203–20.

5. Ingber DE. Tensegrity: the architectural basis of cellular mechanotransduction. Annu Rev Physiol 1997;59:575–99.

6. Janmey PA, Weitz DA. Dealing with mechanics: mechanisms of force transduction in cells. Trends Biochem Sci 2004;29:364–70.

7. Lambert CA, Soudant EP, Lapière CM, et al. Pre-translational regulation of extracellular matrix macromolecules and collagenase expression in fibroblasts by mechanical forces. Lab Invest 1992;66:444–51.

8. Chiquet M. Regulation of extracellular matrix gene expression by mechanical stress. Matrix Biol 1999; 18:417–26.

9. Kessler D, Dethlefsen S, Eckes B, et al. Fibroblasts in mechanically stressed collagen lattices assume a "synthetic" phenotype. J Biol Chem 2001;276: 36575–85.

10. Flück M, Giraud M-N, Chiquet M, et al. Tensile stress-dependent collagen XII and fibronectin production by fibroblasts requires separate pathways. Biochim Biophys Acta 2003;1593:239–48.

11. Bereiter-Hahn J, Lüers H. The role of elasticity in the motile behavior of cells. In: Akkas N, editor. Biomechanics of Active Movement and Division of Cells. Berlin: Springer; 1994. p. 181–230.

12. Fletcher DA, Mullins RD. Cell mechanics and the cytoskeleton. Nature 2010;463:485–92.

13. Kolodney MS, Wysolmerski RB. Isometric contraction by fibroblasts and endothelial cells in tissue culture: a quantitative study. J Cell Biol 1992;117: 73–82.

14. Brown RA, Talas G, Eastwood M, et al. Balanced mechanical forces and microtubule contribution to fibroblast contraction. J Cell Physiol 1996;169:439–47.

15. Uitto J. The role of elastin and collagen in cutaneous aging: intrinsic aging versus photoexposure. J Drugs Dermatol 2008;7(2 Suppl):s12–6.

16. Johnson BD, Page RC, Pieters HP, et al. Effects of donor age on protein and collagen synthesis in vitro by human diploid fibroblasts. Lab Invest 1986;55:490–6.

17. Varani J, Dame MK, Voorhees JJ, et al. Decreased collagen production in chronologically aged skin: roles of age-dependent alteration in fibroblast function and defective mechanical stimulation. Am J Pathol 2006;168:1861–8.

18. Berdyyeva TK, Woodworth CD, Sokolov I. Human epithelial cells increase their rigidity with ageing in vitro: direct measurements. Phys Med Biol 2005; 50:81–92.

19. Sokolov I, Iyer S, Woodworth CD. Recovery of elasticity of aged human epithelial cells in vitro. Nanomedicine 2006;2:31–6.

20. Guck J, Ananthakrishnan R, Käs J, et al. Optical deformability of soft biological dielectrics. Phys Rev Lett 2000;84:5451–4.

21. Guck J, Schinkinger S, Bilby C, et al. Optical deformability as an inherent cell marker for testing malignant transformation and metastatic competence. Biophys J 2005;88:3689–98.

22. Remmerbach TW, Wottawah F, Guck J, et al. Oral cancer diagnosis by mechanical phenotyping. Cancer Res 2009;69:1728–32.

23. Dimri GP, Lee X, Basile G, et al. A biomarker that identifies senescent human cells in culture and in aging skin in vivo. Proc Natl Acad Sci USA 1995; 92:9363–7.

24. Chang E, Harley CB. Telomere length and replicative aging in human vascular tissues. Proc Natl Acad Sci USA 1995;92:11190–4.

25. Herbig U, Ferreira M, Sedivy JM, et al. Cellular senescence in aging primates. Science 2006;311:1257.

26. Collado M, Serrano M. The power and the promise of oncogene-induced senescence markers. Nat Rev Cancer 2006;6:472–6.

27. Kwak IH, Kim HS, Lim IK, et al. Nuclear accumulation of globular actin as a cellular senescence marker. Cancer Res 2004;64:572–80.

28. Janmey PA. Mechanical properties of cytoskeletal polymers. Curr Opin Cell Biol 1991;3:4–11.

29. Rotsch C, Radmacher M. Drug-induced changes of cytoskeletal structure and mechanics in fibroblasts: an atomic force microscopy study. Biophys J 2000; 78:520–35.

30. Grinnell F. Fibroblast-collagen-matrix contraction: growth-factor signalling and mechanical loading. Trends Cell Biol 2000;10:362–5.

31. Walpita D, Hay E. Studying actin-dependent processes in tissue culture. Nat Rev Mol Cell Biol 2002;3:137–41.

32. Petroll WM. Dynamic assessment of cell-matrix mechanical interactions in three-dimensional culture. In: Coutts AS, editor. Methods in Molecular Biology: Adhesion Protein Protocols. 2nd edition. Louisville, KY: Humana; 2007. p. 67–81.

33. Barer R, Joseph S. Refractometry of living cells, Part I. Basic principles. Q J Microsc Sci 1954;95:399–423.

34. Barer R, Joseph S. Refractometry of living cells, Part II. The immersion medium. Q J Microsc Sci 1955a;96:1–26.

35. Barer R, Joseph S. Refractometry of living cells, Part III. Technical and optical methods. Q J Microsc Sci 1955b;96:423–47.

36. Ashkin A. Acceleration and trapping of particles by radiation pressure. Phys Rev Lett 1970;24:156–9.

37. Lincoln B, Wottawah F, Guck J, et al. High-throughput rheological measurements with an optical stretcher. Methods Cell Biol 2007;83:397–423.

38. Wottawah F, Schinkinger S, Käs J, et al. Optical rheology of biological cells. Phys Rev Lett 2005; 94:098103.

39. Holzinger A. Jasplakinolide. An actin-specific reagent that promotes actin polymerization. Methods Mol. Biol 2001;161:109–20.

40. Laudadio RE, Millet EJ, Fredberg JJ, et al. Rat airway smooth muscle cell during actin modulation: rheology and glassy dynamics. Am J Physiol Cell Physiol 2005;289:C1388–95.

41. Gourlay CW, Carpp LN, Ayscough KR, et al. A role for the actin cytoskeleton in cell death and aging in yeast. J Cell Biol 2004;164:803–9.

42. Bubb MR, Spector I, Fosen KM, et al. Effects of jasplakinolide on the kinetics of actin polymerization. An explanation for certain in vivo observations. J Biol Chem 2000;275:5163–70.

43. Knowles GC, McCulloch CAG. Simultaneous localization and quantification of relative G and F actin content: optimization of fluorescence labeling methods. J Histochem Cytochem 1992;40:1605–12.

44. Delvoye P, Wiliquet P, Lapière CM, et al. Measurement of mechanical forces generated by skin fibroblasts embedded in a three-dimensional collagen gel. J Invest Dermatol 1991;97:898–902.

45. Wakatsuki T, Schwab B, Elson EL, et al. Effects of cytochalasin D and latrunculin B on mechanical properties of cells. J Cell Sci 2001;114:1025–36.

46. Rao KM, Cohen HJ. Actin cytoskeletal network in aging and cancer. Mutat Res 1991;256:139–48.

47. Pierard GE, Lapière CM. Physiopathological variations in the mechanical properties of skin. Arch Dermatol Res 1977;260:231–9.

48. Lavker RM, Zheng PS, Dong G. Aged skin: a study by light, transmission electron, and scanning electron microscopy. J Invest Dermatol 1987;88(3 Suppl): 44s–51s.

49. Galli C, Guizzardi S, Scandroglio R, et al. Life on the wire: on tensegrity and force balance in cells. Acta Biomed 2005;76:5–12.

50. Pavalko F, Chen N, Turner C. Fluid shear-induced mechanical signaling in MC3T3–E1 osteoblasts requires cytoskeleton-integrin interactions. Am J Physiol Cell Physiol 1998;275:1591–601.

51. Schneider EL, Mitsui Y. The relationship between in vitro cellular aging and in vivo human age. Proc Natl Acad Sci USA 1976;73:3584–8.

Tissue Engineering of Skin

Fiona Wood

KEYWORDS

- Skin repair • Tissue engineering • Wound healing
- Skin regeneration • Skin development • Scars

INTRODUCTION

Each one of us is a self-organizing mass of multiple cell types. From fertilization of the embryo our tissue structures develop until an adult morphology is achieved. At that point our capacity for self-organization is directed to maintaining that morphology in the face of the insults of our daily life and the processes of aging. When a given insult overwhelms our capacity to repair by regeneration the result is scar repair.[1]

We know that tissues retain a variable ability to heal by regeneration.[2] With respect to the skin, in all but trivial injuries the capacity for regeneration is swamped, triggering the cellular mechanisms which result in scar formation. Burn injury is notorious for aggressive scars, compromising the individual functionally, cosmetically, and psychologically.[3,4]

It has been well described that to heal a wound we need a source of cells capable of differentiation into the given tissue type and an extracellular matrix capable of supporting the cell migration, proliferation, and differentiation.[5] We and others have spent considerable resources researching these areas to improve the speed and quality of wound healing to reduce the scar.[6,7] The question we ask is: "How can we harness the technology of tissue engineering (TE) of skin to provide a controlled repair to restore the original morphology?"

TE can be defined as the application of engineering principles to biological systems.[8] The healing of skin has been the subject of writings back to ancient times with attempts to stimulate healing, protect the surface while healing, and even replace the skin surface.[9] So our recent explorations into using TE principles in skin repair are based on a significant history. With increasing knowledge and understanding of the skin structure and function along with the developing TE techniques can we provide a regenerative repair avoiding scar?

We know that the skin provides the barrier to the external environment as a dynamic, complex three-dimensional structure made up of cells from all embryological layers. Integral to its functions are the vessels and nerves within the cell/matrix construct. Furthermore, skin is specialized over different body sites, adapting to local functional needs demonstrated by the macroscopic differences seen between areas, e.g. the eyelid compared with the palm of hand. The varying capacity to respond to injury is seen with the greater scar potential of sternal and deltoid areas.[10] So as we go forward in developing tissue engineering solutions to skin's it is timely to take stock of the skin functions and interactions. How will the skin changes over the different body sites influence the TE needs? Collaboration with specialists in bioinformatics will be essential in understanding the implication of changes in genes, genetic expression, and the phenotypic expression we need to guide to in the tissue constructs.[11]

In the therapeutic use of TE the understanding of the etiology of the skin defect and pathophysiology of the patient will identify what needs to be replicated, rebuilt, and replaced. Implementation into clinical practice hinges on the TE being problem-driven, providing a practical, timely, cost-effective solution to the clinical problem.[12]

This chapter originally published in *Principles of Regenerative Medicine; Atala A, Lanza R, Thomson JA, Nerem R, 2011, Academic Press, Elsevier, 1063-1078.*

Burns Service of Western Australia, Burn Injury Research Unit, University of Western Australia, McComb Research Foundation, Western Australia
E-mail address: fiona.wood@uwa.edu.au

Clin Plastic Surg 39 (2012) 21–32
doi:10.1016/j.cps.2011.09.004
0094-1298/12/$ – see front matter

TE of skin has developed to this point in response to clinical need of, for example, skin repair in major burns,[13,14] chronic ulcers,[15] and giant nevi.[16] It is clear that the current "gold standard" of skin grafting will always leave a scar.[17] The development of TE gives the opportunity to tailor the repair to the defect with the understanding that one solution will not fit all. TE offers innovative solutions providing a spectrum of clinical solutions from strategies to facilitate wound healing *in situ* to multilayered skin constructs including multiple cell types.

The development of TE of skin is intimately linked to the vision of facilitating scar-free healing.[18] It has broad implications post-trauma, -surgery, and -fibrosing pathologies where the common outcome is a functional compromise due to contracture and loss of normal tissue architecture. In the developed world it is estimated that 100 million patients acquire scars each year, some of which cause considerable problems, as a result of 55 million elective operations and 25 million operations after trauma. Within this number it is estimated that there are in the region of 11 million keloid scars and four million burn scars, 70% of which occur in children.[19]

We are living in a time where science and technology are advancing at an exponential rate. Harnessing the power of that science and technology into clinical practice presents an ever-increasing challenge. We are all aware of the latest breakthrough holding promise to improve the quality of life from the health to the environmental sectors. However, it is worth noting that the exponential growth is possible in controlled systems where experiments can be designed to investigate a single variable; here lies the greatest challenge, for example, in burn injury research. The design of clinical trials is dogged by the complexities of assessing the extent of injury, the individual's response, and the availability of validated outcome measures.

Clinical practice is a fusion of experience and knowledge with the development of medical sub-specialization directed to a targeted problem-solving approach and has facilitated great advances in clinical care. However, this should not be at the expense of a broad general knowledge gaining insight into potential links and facilitating cross-fertilization. It is essential to link the tissue engineer with the clinical specialist to ensure the opportunities, risks, and benefits of TE skin are understood to facilitate appropriate clinical trials. By collaboration between disciplines there are real opportunities for improvements in clinical care translating to improved outcomes for patients.

The road from the bench to the bedside is a long one and navigates the areas of regulation, commercialization, reimbursement, and clinical trial design, to name a few. Also, translational research itself is an area in need of research and audit. The investigation of drivers and barriers to the implementation of TE skin solutions is an area of increasing effort. It is vital to learn from history and understand the current situation to continue developing innovative TE solutions but also innovative solutions within health systems, to action timely translation into clinical practice.

This chapter will:

- explore the functions of the skin and injury responses we need to understand in order to harness the TE technology effectively
- identify the needs which could be supplied by TE strategies
- discuss currently available technologies
- demonstrate TE skin solutions in clinical practice
- highlight the areas of need for further development.

DEVELOPMENT, ANATOMY, AND FUNCTION OF SKIN

Skin is commonly described as a multilayered physical barrier composed chiefly of the surface cellular epidermis and relatively acellular dermis. Exploring the development, anatomy, and skin functions demonstrates its complexity and will guide our TE endeavors.

"There is no magician's mantle to compare with the skin in its diverse roles of waterproof, overcoat, sunshade, suit of armour and refrigerator. Sensitive to the touch of a feather, to temperature and pain, withstanding the wear and tear of three score years and ten and executing its own running repairs."[20]

During development the initial covering of the embryo is the periderm, which is thought to have a barrier function expressing tight junctions and interacts with the amniotic fluid having surface microvilli. It is interesting to note that the periderm cells express keratins also associated with migratory epidermal cells seen in wound healing. During the first 6 weeks the epidermis becomes two-layered, with the outer periderm and the inner developing epidermis. During this time there is no dermis but a subepidermal cellular layer with deposition of basement membrane type IV collagen and laminin by 5 weeks. By 8 weeks there is evidence of vascular development.

During the embryonic fetal transition stage at 9–10 weeks several changes are seen:

- epidermal cells express keratins 1 and 10, associated with differentiation
- maturation of the basement membrane with the development of cell adhesion and expression of integrins α6 and β4
- rapid deposition of dermal matrix
- migration of melanocytes from the neural crest
- Langerhans' cells are detected originating in the fetal thymus and bone marrow
- Merkel cells are seen initially in the epidermis and subsequently in the dermis.

The early fetal period from 11 to 14 weeks sees the development of the hair follicles within the skin. The skin adnexal structures continue to develop and mature into the mid-fetal period at 15–20 weeks. As the fetus grows in the late period, 20–40 weeks, acceleration of stratum corneum can be identified in specific regions, including the palms, soles, face, and scalp. There is a close association between keratinization and hair follicle development with the stratum corneum developing initially in the perifollicular regions. The mature stratum corneum is a structure which develops in the late fetal period; a combination of the terminally differentiated keratinocytes forming a cornified envelope and lipid extrusion from the abundant lamellar bodies of the granular layer keratinocytes.

Embryologically the neural tissue and the epidermis are derived from ectoderm. By the end of the fourth week of embryonic development the neural ectoderm has separated from the surface ectoderm forming the neural tube. The nerve endings will never, under normal conditions, be exposed to the external environment. The skin forms the interface and has developed as the interactive responsive surface. In the following weeks mesoblastic cells from the neural crest migrate into the skin as melanoblasts and the early nerve fibers develop as the vasculature migrates into the mesodermal elements destined to become dermis. A close association is seen in development with the skin, developing as a tactile organ providing the feedback information from the surface to the developing CNS. The understanding of neural plasticity of the CNS and the peripheral nerve field underpins the self-organization principle. The co-development is put forward as an explanation of the co-evolution of the human CNS and the skin as an adaptive dynamic interface.

In the fully developed skin there are cells from all three embryological layers in a complex framework of extracellular matrix (ECM). There are functions common to all skin areas, but also there has been adaptation to the specific functions of given body sites which are seen even at the early fetal stages.

The mature epidermis is composed primarily of keratinocytes arising from a layer of basal cells situated on the basement membrane. As the keratinocytes differentiate they form a stratified squamous epithelium. As the cells undergo terminal differentiation they lose their nuclei and form a highly cross-linked protein-based layer of keratin. The basal cells are in intimate contact with terminal dendrites: synapse-like structures have been described between nerve endings and keratinocytes. The melanocytes are situated in the basal layer with the melanosomes being transferred to the differentiating keratinocytes giving the color of the skin due to pigment load. The cells linking to the immune system, Langerhans' giant cells and dendritic cells, are also present in the epidermis. The epidermis is specialized to the body sites, most noticeably with the thickened cornified layer of the sole and palm.

The dermis is attached to the epidermis at the dermal–epidermal junction by the basement membrane morphologically arranged as the rete pegs, which are exaggerated at glaberous skin areas. The dermis is mainly connective tissue, predominantly collagen, with elastin seen in the superficial papillary dermis. The fibroblast is the cell that produces the ECM, which is specialized over differing body sites with areas such as the groin and axilla being more elastic thanthe thicker dermis of the back. Cells of hematopoietic origin such as lymphoctyes and macrophages migrate into the dermis and are involved in surveillance. The neural and vascular networks maintain the skin and facilitate the functions of the dynamic interactive skin interface.[21]

The investigation of wound healing in parallel with an understanding of skin development and functions gives us the opportunity to further develop innovative methods of TE. The skin has developed specifically in relation to the multiple functions it performs. As an active organ it is responsive to changes in the external and internal environment, pivotal in maintaining the body's homeostasis. Our knowledge of skin functions is still growing and includes:

- semi-permeable barrier, overcoat, suit of armor
- thermoregulation, refrigerator
- antibacterial, waterproof
- UV protection, sunshade

- sensory receptor, sensitive to the touch of a feather, to temperature, and to pain
- self-regenerating, withstanding the wear and tear of a lifetime
- capable of rapid repair, executing its own running repairs
- immune modulation
- psychological interaction
- vitamin production.

The loss of skin integrity can result in severe morbidity and even mortality. The body needs a barrier to the atmosphere to maintain homeostasis. The production of the stratum corneum can be mimicked in tissue culture by exposing a sheet of keratinocytes in culture to an air–liquid interface,[22] but it requires maturation in situ to fully develop the "smart material" of the anucleated cell bodies and the extracellular lipoproteins moisturized by vitamin E-producing sebum.

The keratinocytes produce surface proteins which are antimicrobial in the first line of defense against the colonizing bacteria on the skin surface.[23] The expression of these proteins changes as the keratinocyte is stressed, as in wounding or culturing, such that protection from microbial invasion is highlighted.

The multiple and specific sensory inputs to the skin are pivotal in the regulation of the body's temperature, immune responses, and the psychological responses via neural and neuroendocrine control systems. Recent animal studies have highlighted the sensory role of the skin in normal development, with touch being associated with growth potential of the internal solid organs.[21]

The skin is also profoundly influenced by the pathophysiology of the individual, with cutaneous changes in anatomy and physiology being linked to many disease processes.

It is with this expanding body of knowledge with respect to the skin that we engage the fields of TE to provide solutions for skin defects to maintain function and avoid scarring. To do so we also need a working knowledge of the skin response to injury and tissue loss; the processes of wound healing.

Briefly, wound healing in skin is a complex series of cascading events which has been described in three overlapping stages from the initial inflammation to tissue formation and subsequent tissue remodeling.[24,25]

The initial response is clot formation to achieve hemostasis. The activation of platelets releases the contents of their alpha granules, resulting in the activation of the clotting cascade and the release of adhesive proteins forming the matrix of the clot, e.g. fibrin and chemotactic factors and growth factors into the wounded area. The coagulation pathway links to the activation of the complement pathway's facilitation of the recruitment of neutrophils needed to facilitate the inflammatory response with the removal of cellular debris and microorganisms.

The in-growth of new vessels as granulation tissue is initiated and the keratinocytes at the wound edge mobilize to commence re-epithelialization. Macrophages migrate to the wound, releasing multiple protein growth factors as the wound response progresses to the repair phase. Both hemopoietic and mesenchymal stem cells from the circulation are attracted into the wound with fibroblasts producing ECM, some as myofibroblasts associated with wound contraction.

There is an increased interest in the interactions between the keratinocytes and underlying fibroblasts as the matrix is remodeled and the new basement membrane develops. As the keratinocyte is exposed to collagen it secretes collagenase and as the basement membrane integrity is restored the cells revert to their normal phenotype in the situation where healing is achieved without scarring.

In situations of more extensive tissue damage the fibroblast is of a scar phenotype with the production of disordered collagen. The interactions between the ECM and the fibroblasts respond to the changes as healing progresses from tissue repair to remodeling. The initial migratory fibroblast transitions to the profibrotic phenotype producing ECM proteins. In the remodeling phase the cell number within the dermis or scar falls as the cells undergo apoptosis.

A knowledge of the wound-healing progression over time allows the TE skin solution to be clinically integrated into the process and may be directed at a number of target strategies: the control of cells in growth, the genetic manipulation of cells to express a given phenotype, seeding of the retained dermis with cells from the dermal–epidermal junction, removal of the full thickness of the area of compromised skin, and replacement with a TE construct.

THE POTENTIAL PREREQUISITE REQUIREMENTS FOR TE SKIN SOLUTIONS

The skin matures from the softness of the newborn to the skin in old age with the loss of elasticity.[26] We believe that the young heal rapidly but scar aggressively, in contrast to the elderly, who heal more slowly and scar less. Regeneration of the skin without functional or aesthetic deficit, rather than enhanced repair, remains the ultimate goal of wound healing therapies.[27] However, the degree of scarring and the quality of the repair are highly dependent on the time taken to heal, with faster healing correlating to improved outcome.[6] The availability of the TE skin for timely use is a key factor balancing the issues of allograft to autograft, biological to non-biological solutions. The differences in wound healing responses with age and etiology of the defect will have implications when harvesting donor tissue for TE and will potentially influence the choice of TE technique.[28]

The skin surface is continually replaced under normal conditions and the morphology is retained over the years. However, the capacity to regenerate and self-organize becomes overwhelmed in all but trivial injuries such that the repair forms a scar which all too often is debilitating, both physically and psychologically. The traditional approach to reduce the time to healing of a skin defect has been to skin graft. Full-thickness skin grafts (FTG) will give the best scar result but appropriate donor sites to match with recipient sites can lead to skin mismatch, as seen when a FTG from the groin is used to release a contracture on the palm of the hand. The donor site availability for split-thickness skin grafting (SSG) may be limited in size when large body surface areas are compromised as in burn injury or giant nevi. The area of cover of a given donor site can be increased by meshing or expanding as in the Meek technique.[29] The expansion of the SSG is associated with small areas of the wound healing by secondary intention and a poorer scar outcome. It is the desire to eliminate, or at least reduce the scar with reduction of donor site morbidity, that has driven TE of skin over the last three decades.

The essential factors to achieve healing are:

- a source of cell's capable of differentiating into the tissue
- an extracellular matrix capable of supporting the cells.

With an increased understanding of the skin physiology and interactions with the internal and external environment we need to also consider:

- the three-dimensional spacial information of the area under repair
- feedback from the surface to facilitate self-organization.

The ideal needs for a TE skin replacement continue to be debated and are related to the clinical indication for use. In our group we have been guided by the following basic requirements[30]:

- rapidly available
- autologous
- site-matched
- reliable wound adherence
- minimal donor site morbidity
- clinically manageable
- improved quality of scar
- affordable.

For TE to be successful it is clear that an in-depth working knowledge of the biology of the tissue is essential. There are a number of cell types within the skin, each with specific and often inter-related functions; it is fundamental to the success of TE to have an understanding of the essential information on how the cells relate to the other cells and the ECM of the skin.

The ECM scaffold is integral to tissue integrity, we know that the physical shape and chemical composition of the environment of a cell influence its phenotype. The field of bioinformatics may well assist in refining design in the future.[31] In the design of the TE solution the understanding of this relationship will lead to increased clinical success.

From the engineering perspective there are technologies which will facilitate innovative clinical solutions such as the advanced modeling and fabrication for scaffold manufacture. The development of bioreactors to maintain viability and expand cell numbers associated with scale up in an appropriately regulated laboratory is essential for cell-culture-based techniques.[22]

It is also clear from the experiences of the last three decades that many of the proposed TE skin solutions are disruptive technologies. It is essential that the TE skin should not only be designed for a clinical problem, be reproducible and reliable, but also be linked to an education and training program such that it realizes its full clinical potential.

CURRENT TE SKIN TECHNOLOGIES

Engineering principles have been applied to skin for many years with the development of medical devices to harvest SSG accurately and mesh the skin to allow expansion. The practice of tissue expansion is a well-established surgical tool for the development of skin by subcutaneous insertion of inflatable devices *in vivo*, which can be serially enlarged with the resulting development of the skin as demonstrated by cell proliferation.[32] The tissue-expanded skin has all layers and the complete characteristics of the donor site including retention of functional innervation.[33] There is an increasing interest in the concept of tissue expansion *in vitro* with a full-thickness skin biopsy put under tension in a bioreactor system to maintain its viability and facilitate cell replication resulting in tissue growth. However, these solutions are limited by time, area, and in some cases donor site and scar outcome. There remains the need to provide rapid large surface area cover with the ultimate goal of healing by regeneration, not scar repair.

The initial approach to TE skin was to separate the layers and consider the epidermis and dermis as separate problems.

The work by Green in the 1970s was focused on the culture of keratinocytes into cell sheets suitable for grafting.[34] The solution to the large surface area burn was to harvest cells from a non-injured donor site and undertake laboratory-based tissue expansion. The resulting sheets of cells could be used to close the wound as would a traditional SSG. However, there were problems with the time taken to culture in the laboratory, fragility, adherence to the wound surface, and durability over time as only the epidermis was replaced, in addition to the cost.[13,14] In trying to solve some of these problems there has been development in the area of subconfluent cell transfer on a number of cell culture surfaces[35] in addition to the delivery of cells in suspension as an aerosol.[36,37] The subconfluent cells have a more reliable adherence and are available in a shorter timeframe from 3 weeks for sheets to 5 days for subconfluent cultures.[38,39] The process of harvesting cells from the dermal–epidermal junction by enzymatic and physical dissociation has been used for immediate delivery of a non-cultured cell population to the wound.[40] The cells are a mixed cell population in the same ratio as seen in the normal skin construct as there has been no selection of cell populations seen when culturing. The maintenance of the melanocytes allows the development of appropriate pigmentation.[41] The cells adhere, migrate, and proliferate across the wound surface and then differentiate and self-organize into a mature epidermis. The scar outcome is intimately linked to the underlying wound bed, which will be discussed in a later section.

The development of a suitable dermal scaffold was also the focus of the TE field.[42] Topographical features are known to influence cell behavior through a phenomenon known as "contact guidance," and alteration in the size of the surface detail can elicit different cell responses.[43] Running parallel to the epidermal cell culture was work by Yannas and Burke on dermal replacement, which culminated in the commercially available product Integra.[44] The concept of tissue-guided regeneration within an architectural framework is in current clinical practice. The underpinning research on the composition and construction demonstrated the importance of considering both aspects; a combination of bovine collagen coated with GAG but with a pore size of less than 60 µm or greater than 100 µm resulting in disordered granulation tissue, with the optimal pore size resulting in the migrating cells expressing a reticular dermal fibroblast phenotype. The main drawback with Integra is that is addresses only the dermal aspect, with the outer layer on silicone acting as a pseudo-epidermis for the period on vascularization, usually 3 weeks before a second surgical procedure is needed to repair the epidermis.[45] The epidermal repair is with a thin SSG which may be meshed to cover a larger area than the donor site with epidermal cells to speed the time to healing and reduce the mesh scar pattern.[46] The two-stage problem has been addressed by trying to reduce the time to vascularization or by the development of constructs that can be used with an SSG at the same procedure; Apligraft, Matriderm, and Pelnec are dermal templates marketed to provide appropriate topography and matrix properties to promote cell migration into the wound, improve healing, and reduce scarring as a one-stage procedure with SSG.[47] An alternative is to use our knowledge of healing as we see cells migrating from areas of the skin adnexal structures in the dermis to form the new epidermal layer; introduced cells harvested from the dermal–epidermal junction seeded into the Integra will migrate and organize into a new epidermis with an established dermal–epidermal junction within 3 weeks.[48] The use of Integra is a clear demonstration of the potential of tissue-guided regeneration with the expression of cell phenotype guided by the morphology and chemistry of the matrix.[49]

It is well established that cells change their phenotype in response to changes in their environment.[50,51] The development of suitable technologies to generate an optimal environment for wound healing is key to enhancing cell response to tissue injury, reducing the time to heal and improving the outcome. Our knowledge of the ECM–cell interactions is increasing with the recognition of the cell signaling by nanoscale structures on cell surfaces with roles in attachment and cell migration.[52] Developments in nanotechnology have opened up possibilities in TE to improve on scaffold design, but relatively little is known about how changes in topography at the nanoscale affect cell behavior.[53] The scaffolds can be manufactured to address specific skin functions: to protect the injury from loss of fluid and proteins, enable the removal of exudates, inhibiting exogenous microorganism invasion, and improve the aesthetic appearance of the wound site.[54] Current scaffolds are generally matrices of synthetic and/ or natural polymers, fabricated by various techniques including[55] solvent-casting, gas foaming, electrospinning, phase separation, freeze drying, melt molding, and solid free-form fabrication.[56] Key to their performance is reproducibility, with control over pore size and the distribution of pores, removal of residual toxic organic solvents, and the control of the inflammatory and immune responses due to polymer degradation and the associated by-products.[57]

Our group has explored anodic aluminum oxide (AAO) as a potential scaffold or template in TE.[58] The self-organized oxide growth under controlled conditions generates a densely packed hexagonal array of uniform-size nanopores aligned perpendicular to the surface of the AAO film. The size of the pores can be nanoengineered by manipulating the anodization time and voltage, the anodizing electrolyte, and/or the time of post-chemical etching. Aluminum oxide is well known for its biocompatibility in the human body; it is inert, stable, and non-reactive, making it suitable for TE applications. The engineering of surfaces to manipulate healing is a rapidly expanding area, with the use of interactive dressing systems in widespread clinical use. With the realization of the impact of surface topography and chemistry on cell expression, and the developing nanoengineering techniques such as electrospinning and electrospraying, there is increasing interest in smart surface technology skin healing. Biocompatible polymeric self-assembling nanofiber constructs have the advantage of a large surface area, which can be linked to bioactive compounds. The release of the bioactive compounds can be controlled by intrinsic factors such as, in a hydrogel, release kinetics or extrinsic release triggers.[59] Recent exciting advances have been made in the area of nanocubes, nanocages, and nanorods, as primary candidates to be studied for the phototherapeutic release of bioactive agents.[60] Clinically, the results of single cytokine applications have been disappointing and study of the natural healing processes is a result of complex cascade interactions over time.[61] It should be hardly surprising that we cannot achieve with a single cytokine administration what is the result of cell–ECM interactions. The aim with the advancing technology is to mimic the structure and function of the ECM, with the ability to adapt over time to the changing environment of the healing wound.[62]

Bringing together the scaffold and cellular components has been successful with the development of multilayered constructs seeded with multiple cell types.[27,63] Clinical series have been presented demonstrating a soft supple skin but with the persistent problem of poor color match.[64] The understanding of the interdependence of the cells of the dermal–epidermal junction may well be key in the development of skin constructs with the appropriate melanocyte function.[65] The main drawback in the clinical use of complex laboratory-based constructs is the time taken in the laboratory.[66] However, the potential to use such technology in timed reconstructive surgery as opposed to acute trauma is beneficial with the ability to tailor the skin construct to the planned defect. The three-dimensional distribution of cells within the wound has been addressed by the innovative use of the "ink jet printing" technology, with the cells "printed," controlled by the shape and depth of the defect. The cell type within the system can be changed with the fibroblasts being laid down prior to the keratinocytes.[67] ECM and other proteins can also be introduced into the system, such as hair-based keratins, chemical-processing substrates from biological origins to develop innovative scaffold solutions to enhance cell performance within the constructs.

The time to availability of a TE technique is a key driver to the clinical utilization.[68] The use of allograft materials allows an "off the shelf" approach, whereas autograft material may take time in the expansion phase. The use of scaffolds alone can provide an advanced wound management system to facilitate healing, and can replace a tissue defect guiding repair as it is replaced or provide a permanent solution. The use of cells alone can also provide a surface epithelium which can modulate the underlying healing, form a mosaic of cells of intrinsic and extrinsic origin guiding repair, or provide a permanent surface. The combination of the two elements can provide an advanced skin repair solution, but as the differentiation of the construct is more advanced the time taken in the processes is prolonged. Consideration of the time taken has led to the investigation of construct being used in the immature form differentiating in situ. It is clear that TE provides a range of innovative solutions which are useful in a range of wounding/skin replacement areas. The effective use of the technology hinges on the clinician understanding the wound preparation and the aim of the repair. The wound assessment drives the initial clinical decisions directing management in terms of resuscitation, tissue salvage, infection control, and then planning the repair. The understanding of the range of

TE solutions is essential in appropriate clinical implementation.

TE SKIN SOLUTIONS IN CLINICAL PRACTICE

The following clinical case of an extensive 65% total body surface area (TBSA) burn injury associated with multiple fractures and pneumothorax is used to demonstrate the decision-making and options available in current practice. The initial stabilization and resuscitation is life-saving, along with attention to infection control using Acticoat, a nanocrystalline silver dressing. Once stable, surgical debridement is planned to excise the areas of skin which cannot be salvaged. Although the timing of debridement is vigorously debated with respect to controlling the ongoing inflammation and improving outcome potential, a key element in the decision-making is what is available to cover the debrided wounds, either as a temporary measure or as a permanent replacement. A full-thickness wound requires dermal and epidermal repair for the optimal outcome. In large-surface-area wounds the standard SSG is not possible in one procedure due to restricted donor sites; the SSG can be meshed to achieve healing in a larger area but the healing of the interstices by secondary intention often leaves an unsightly meshed pattern scar. Cadaver allograft has been widely used but provides only a temporary solution and will require serial cover as the donor sites heal. A combination of allograft dermis and sheet cultured epithelial autograft (CEA) has been reported to result in a composite repair with retention of the dermal elements. The CEA sheets may take 21 days to culture, or more timely availability can be achieved using preconfluent cultures on carriers or delivered as suspension. The dermis can be replaced now with a number of off-the-shelf products such as Matriderm, Pelnec, or Apligraft. The TE technique most widely reported to date is Integra. The use of composite TE skin could be considered to augment the second stage of the repair with Integra, as it takes time in laboratory preparation.

In this case Integra was used to reconstruct the dermis in the areas of full-thickness excision, as seen in **Fig. 1**, where the Integra is held in place with a combination of staples and dressings to facilitate take. In areas where dermis could be salvaged cells were harvested from the dermal–epidermal junction of uninjured skin using a ReCell kit with Biobrane as a dressing. The main drawback with Integra is the period of vascularization of 3 weeks prior to proceeding to repair of the epidermis. The epidermis was repaired using a thin meshed SSG 1 to 3 in combination with

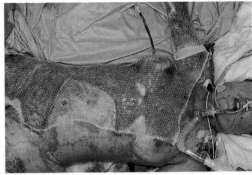

Fig. 1. Post-surgical debridement of full-thickness burn of 65% TBSA and replacement with Integra dermal scaffold held in place with Fastinet, area of partial-thickness burn on the abdomen treated with autologous cells under Biobrane, and non-injured skin donor site on the left flank.

a non-cultured cell suspension from the ReCell kit to reduce the meshed pattern scar. The healing is seen in **Fig. 2** with the mash pattern fading well in the upper compared to the lower abdomen. At the time of scar maturity in **Fig. 3**, the scar situation demonstrates the current issues faced by our patients:

- contour deflect due to removed subcutaneous fat layer
- persistent mesh pattern in the lower scar
- mismatch of pigmentation
- contracture bands distorting the anatomy
- the repair is a scar.

There has clearly been progress with the development of TE techniques intimately linked with the advancing survival and quality of scar in patients with major burn injuries. However, there is a clear need to continue to develop TE with the aim of total three-dimensional soft tissue and skin replacement.

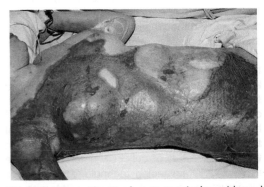

Fig. 2. Post second procedure to repair the epidermal layer using a combination of meshed split-thickness graft with a non-cultured autologous cell spray.

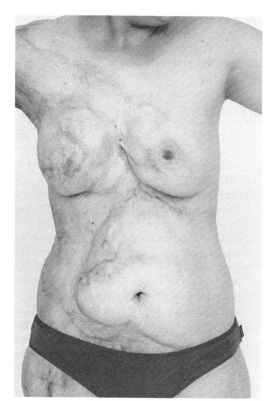

Fig. 3. Two years post-injury, prior to planned reconstructive surgery.

THE FUTURE

It is the vision of scarless healing which has led to the exploration of regeneration and the interplay between genes,[69] cells, and tissues. Pleuripotential stem cells are present within each individual; the drivers of the cells down a regenerative path are as yet unknown but an exciting area of research with promise for the future.[70] The introduction of allograft stem cells such as mesenchymal stem cells may provide an alternative source of cell regeneration.[71] Understanding that every intervention from the time of injury influences the scar worn for life has driven research in a multitude of directions. TE of skin is an exciting area which already has made a significant clinical impact.[72] However, we are far from the routine provision of technologies and strategies to provide site-matched fully functional skin.[73] Great progress has been made in the areas of dermal templates and cell-based therapies and bringing the two elements together in skin constructs. The clinical implementation of TE skin solutions, along with the use of interactive surface dressing systems, has improved outcomes.

The task is far from completed:

- skin adnexal structures are elusive
- timely availability of TE skin remains problematic

and more work is needed in:

- harnessing the explosion in smart material technology
- understanding the drivers to tissue-guided regeneration
- understanding the concept of self-organization and the bioinformatics behind morphology
- investigating the impact of neural plasticity and its role in scarless healing
- understanding the barriers to clinical translation
- developing regulatory pathways for novel solutions to ensure safety but timely availability.

At the high-tech end of the spectrum we may consider bringing together laser surface imaging linked to fabrication to build bioreactors the shape of the defect with the "smart" cytokine-loaded scaffold materials tailored to the correct three-dimensional shape. Cells of the appropriate body site could then be introduced into the scaffold by cell printing methods in the individualized bioreactor and flow of tissue culture medium used to induce small-vessel formation. At the time of transplant application of external techniques such as infrared could control the release of biologically active molecules from the "smart" scaffold surface to ensure, for instance, reinnervation and restoration of function with the capacity to integrate into the body. An alternative to the individualized bioreactor could be the wound itself prepared by "smart" surface sand seeded with cells directly. With the understanding of the drivers to self-organization they could be used to enhance *in situ* tissue-guided regeneration.

SUMMARY

Over the last three decades the concept of TE has been an area of active research, investigating innovative solutions. Combinations of three-dimensonal engineered scaffolds with cells to produce tissue over time provide the fourth dimension of skin repair techniques.

The fundamental elements required for primary healing are:

- a source of cells capable of differentiation into the lost tissue

- an architectural framework for cells to migrate into and express the appropriate phenotype
- three-dimensional spatial information of the damaged tissue and the relationship to the surrounding viable non-injured tissue interface
- a feedback mechanism to guide self-organization.

In July 2005 the *Medical Journal of Australia* published a vision of clinical care in a number of disciplines in 50 years' time.

> "*Assessment* is key in understanding the extent of injury.
> *Debridement* is focused on tissue salvage.
> *Reconstruction* balances repair with regeneration.
> Investigation of multimodality, multiscale characterisation, including confocal microscopy and synchrotron technology will quantify assessment.
> *Debridement* using autolytic inflammatory control techniques with image guided physical methods will ensure the vital tissue frameworks are retained.
> Tissue guided regeneration afforded by self-assembly nano-particles will provide the framework to guide cells to express the appropriate phenotype in *reconstruction*.
> To solve the clinical problem a multidisciplinary scientific approach is needed to ensure the quality of the scar is worth the pain of survival."

It is of note that already many of the technologies highlighted are available and in need of research to move along the innovation pathway to ensure safe implementation into healthcare systems. Progress requires collaboration at all stages from basic science, clinical trial design to health economics, driven by improved clinical outcomes. Translation of new technologies into health systems requires the rigor of a research framework to identify and measure the impact of innovation in communication and education. Close working relationships between basic research and clinical service delivery are essential.

If the solution to the problem is scarless healing by a regenerative repair process and the aim is to improve the outcome from injury by restoration of function, then the future must blend the long-term vision with incremental short-term improvements.

There has been great progress in TE of skin to date, and it is an exciting area which offers tangible clinical solutions with an enormous potential for further improvement. The challenge we face now is to capitalize on that tradition and link with the opportunities afforded by the unprecedented growth in science and technology, to ensure the quality of the scar outcome is worth the pain of survival.

REFERENCES

1. Ferguson MW, O'Kane S. Scar-free healing: from embryonic mechanisms to adult therapeutic intervention. Philos Trans R Soc Lond B Biol Sci 2004;359:839–50.
2. Martinez-Hernandez A. Repair, regeneration, and fibrosis. In: Rubin E, Farber JL, editors. Pathology. Philadelphia: J B Lippincott; 1988. p. 66–95.
3. Rockwell WB, Cohen IK, Ehrlich HP. Keloids and hypertrophic scars: a comprehensive review. Plast Reconstr Surg 1989;84:827–37.
4. Rumsey N, Clarke A, White P. Exploring the psychosocial concerns of outpatients with disfiguring conditions. J Wound Care 2003;12:247–52.
5. Bannasch H, Fohn M, Unterberg T, et al. Skin tissue engineering. Clin Plast Surg 2003;30:573–9.
6. Deitch EA, Wheelahan TM, Rose MP, et al. Hypertrophic burn scars: analysis of variables. J Trauma 1983;23:895–8.
7. Wood FM. Clinical potential of cellular autologous epithelial suspension. Wounds 2003;15:16–22.
8. Johnson PC, Mikos CG, Fisher JP, et al. Strategic directions in tissue engineering. Tissue Eng 2007; 13:2827–37.
9. Roupé KM, Nybo M, Sjöbring U, et al. Injury is a major inducer of epidermal innate immune responses during wound healing. J Invest Dermatol 2010;130:910–6.
10. Mustoe TA, Cooter RD, Gold MH, et al. International clinical recommendations on scar management. Plast Reconstr Surg 2002;110:560–71.
11. Smiley AK, Klingenberg JM, Aronow BJ, et al. Microarray analysis of gene expression in cultured skin substitutes compared with native human skin. J Invest Dermatol 2005;125:1286–301.
12. Shakespeare P, Shakespeare V. Survey: use of skin substitute materials in UK burn treatment centres. Burns 2002;28:295–7.
13. Wood FM, Kolybaba ML, Allen P. The use of cultured epithelial autograft in the treatment of major burn injuries: a critical review of the literature. Burns 2006;32:395–401.
14. Wood FM, Kolybaba ML, Allen P. The use of cultured epithelial autograft in the treatment of major burn wounds: eleven years of clinical experience. Burns 2006;32:538–44.
15. Llames SG, Del Rio M, Larcher F, et al. Human plasma as a dermal scaffold for the generation of a completely autologous bioengineered skin. Transplantation 2004;77:350–5.

16. Whang K, Kim M, Song W, et al. Comparative treatment of giant congenital melanocytic nevi with curettage or Er:YAG laser ablation alone versus with cultured epithelial autografts. Dermatol Surg 2005;31:1660–7.

17. Mosier MJ, Gibran NS. Surgical excision of the burn wound. Clin Plastic Surg 2009;36:617–25.

18. Atiyeh BS, Costagliola M. Cultured epithelial autograft (CEA) in burn treatment: three decades later. Burns 2007;33:405–13.

19. Bayat A. Skin scarring. BMJ 2003;326:88–92.

20. Lockhart RD, Hamilton GF, Fyfe FW. Anatomy of the Human Body. Philadelphia: J B Lippincott; 1965.

21. Hoath SB, Maibach HI. Neonatal Skin: Structure and Function. New York: Marcel Dekker; 2003.

22. Kalyanaraman B, Boyce S. Assessment of an automated bioreactor to propagate and harvest keratinocytes for fabrication of engineered skin substitutes. Tissue Eng 2007;13:983–93.

23. Bardan A, Nizet V, Gallo RL. Antimicrobial peptides and the skin. Expert Opin Biol Ther 2004;4:543–9.

24. Greenhalgh DG. Models of wound care. J Burn Care Rehabil 2005;26:293–395.

25. Singer AJ, Clark RA. Cutaneous wound healing. N Engl J Med 1999;341:738–46.

26. Fuchs E. Scratching the surface of skin development. Nature 2007;445:834–42.

27. Boyce ST. Design principles for composition and performance of cultured skin substitutes. Burns 2001;27:523–33.

28. Horch RE, Kopp J, Kneser U, et al. Tissue engineering of cultured skin substitutes. J Cell Mol Med 2005;9:592–608.

29. Munster AM, Smith-Meek M. The effect of early surgical intervention on mortality and cost effectiveness in burn care 1978–1991. Burns 1994;20:61–4.

30. Martin P. Wound healing—aiming for perfect skin regeneration. Science 1997;276:75–81.

31. Powell HM, McFarland KL, Butler DL, et al. Uniaxial strain regulates morphogenesis, gene expression, and tissue strength in engineered skin. Tissue Eng Part A 2010;16:1083–92.

32. Argenta LC. Controlled tissue expansion in reconstructive surgery. Br J Plast Surg 1984;37:520–6.

33. Wood FM, McMahon SB. The response of the peripheral nerve field to controlled soft tissue expansion. Br J Plast Surg 1989;42:682–6.

34. Rheinwald JG, Green H. Serial cultivation of strains of human epidermal keratinocytes: the formation of keratinizing colonies from single cells. Cell 1975;6:331–43.

35. Chester DL, Balderson DS, Papini RP. A review of keratinocyte delivery to the wound bed. J Burn Care Rehabil 2004;25:266–75.

36. Currie LJ, Martin R, Sharpe JR, et al. A comparison of keratinocyte cell sprays with and without fibrin glue. Burns 2003;29:677–85.

37. Fredriksson C, Kratz G, Huss F. Transplantation of cultured human keratinocytes in single cell suspension: a comparative in vitro study of different application techniques. Burns 2008;34:212–9.

38. Hernon CA, Dawson RA, Freedlander E, et al. Clinical experience using cultured epithelial autografts leads to an alternative methodology for transferring skin cells from the laboratory to the patient. Regen Med 2006;1:809–21.

39. Johnen C, Steffen I, Beichelt D, et al. Culture of subconfluent human fibroblasts and keratinocytes using biodegradable transfer membranes. Burns 2008;34:655–63.

40. Wood F. Alternative delivery of keratinocytes for epidermal replacement. In: Orgill DP, Blanco C, Joseph M, editors. Biomaterials for Treating Skin Loss. Cambridge: Woodhead Publishing; 2008.

41. Navarro FA, Stoner ML, Lee HB, et al. Melanocyte repopulation in full-thickness wounds using a cell spray apparatus. J Burn Care Rehabil 2001;22:41–6.

42. Klama-Baryła A, Glik J, Kawecki M, et al. Skin substitutes–the application of tissue engineering in burn treatment Part 1. J Orthop Trauma Sur Rel Res 2008;3:96–103.

43. Freytes DO, Wan LQ, Vunjak-Novakovic G. Geometry and force control of cell function. J Cell Biochem 2009;108:1047–58.

44. Yannas IV, Burke JF, Huang C, et al. Correlation of in vivo collagen degradation rate with in vitro measurements. J Biomed Mater Res 1975;9:623–8.

45. Heitland A, Piatkowski A, Noah EM, et al. Update on the use of collagen/glycosaminoglycate skin substitute – six years of experiences with artificial skin in 15 German burn centers. Burns 2004;30:471–5.

46. Navarro FA, Stoner ML, Parks CS, et al. Sprayed keratinocyte suspensions accelerate epidernal coverage in porcine microwound model. J Burn Care Rehabil 2000;21:513–8.

47. Bannasch H, Unterberg T, Fohn M, et al. Cultured keratinocytes in fibrin with decellularised dermis close porcine full-thickness wounds in a single step. Burns 2008;34:1015–20.

48. Wood FM, Stoner ML, Fowler BV, et al. The use of a non-cultured autologous cell suspension and Integra dermal regeneration template to repair full-thickness skin wounds in a porcine model: a one-step process. Burns 2007;33:693–700.

49. Orgill DP, Straus FH II, Lee RC. The use of collagen-GAG membranes in reconstructive surgery. Ann N Y Acad Sci 1999;888:233–48.

50. Smiley AK, Klingenberg JM, Boyce ST, et al. Keratin expression in cultured skin substitutes suggests that the hyperproliferative phenotype observed in vitro is normalized after grafting. Burns 2006;32:135–8.

51. Takahashi K, Yamanaka S. Induction of pluripotent stem cells from mouse embryonic an adult fibroblast cultures by defined factors. Cell 2006;126:663–76.

52. Black AF, Bouez C, Perrier E, et al. Optimization and characterization of an engineered human skin equivalent. Tissue Eng 2005;11:723–33.

53. Fleming RG, Murphy CJ, Abrams GA, et al. Effects of synthetic micro- and nano-structured surfaces on cell behaviour. Biomaterials 1999;20:573–88.

54. Curtis A, Wilkinson C. Nantotechniques and approaches in biotechnology. Trends Biotechnol 2001;19:97–101.

55. Wilkinson CDW, Riehle M, Wood M, et al. The use of materials patterned on a nano- and micro-metric scale in cellular engineering. Mater Sci Eng C 2002;19:263–9.

56. Smith LA, Ma PX. Nano-fibrous scaffolds for tissue engineering. Colloid Surfaces B: Biointerfaces 2004;39:125–31.

57. Chin SF, Iyer KS, Saunders M, et al. Encapsulation and sustained release of curcumin using super-paramagnetic silica reservoirs. Chem Eur J 2009;15:5661–9.

58. Parkinson LG, Giles NL, Adcroft KF, et al. The potential of nanoporous anodic aluminium oxide membranes to influence skin wound repair. Tissue Eng Part A 2009;15:3753–6.

59. Yamato M. Cell sheet engineering: from temperature-responsive culture surfaces to clinics. Eur Cell Mater 2003;6:420–8.

60. Nath N, Hyun J. Surface engineering strategies for control of protein and cell interactions. Surface Sci 2004;570:98–110.

61. Eppley BL, Woodell JE, Higgins J. Platelet quantification and growth factor analysis from platelet-rich plasma: implications for wound healing. Plast Reconstr Surg 2003;114:1502–8.

62. Liu H, Mao J, Yao K, et al. A study on a chitosan-gelatin-hyaluronic acid scaffold as artificial skin *in vitro* and its tissue engineering applications. J Biomater Sci Polym Ed 2004;15:25–40.

63. Sheridan RL, Morgan JR, Cusick JL, et al. Initial experience with a composite autologous skin substitute. Burns 2001;27:421–4.

64. Boyce ST, Kagan RJ, Greenhalgh DG, et al. Cultured skin substitutes reduce requirements for harvesting of skin autograft for closure of excised, full-thickness burns. J Trauma 2006;60:821–9.

65. Mizoguchi M, Suga Y, Sanmano B, et al. Organo-typic culture and surface plantation using umbilical cord epithelial cells: morphogenesis and expression of differentiation markers mimicking cutaneous epidermis. J Dermatol Sci 2004;35:199–220.

66. Meana A, Iglesias J, Del Rio M, et al. Large surface of cultured human epithelium obtained on a dermal matrix based on live fibroblast-containing fibrin gels. Burns 1998;24:621–30.

67. Lamme EN, Van Leeuwen RT, Brandsma K, et al. Higher numbers of autologous fibroblasts in an artificial dermal substitute improve tissue regeneration and modulate scar tissue formation. J Pathol 2000;190:595–603.

68. Carsin H, Ainaud P, Le Bever H, et al. Cultured epithelial autografts in extensive burn coverage of severely traumatized patients: a five year single-center experience with 30 patients. Burns 2000;26:379–87.

69. Goessler UR, Riedel K, Hormann K, et al. Perspectives of gene therapy in stem cell tissue engineering. Cells Tissues Organs 2006;183:169–79.

70. Madlambayan G, Rogers I. Umbilical cord-derived stem cells for tissue therapy: current and future uses. Regen Med 2006;1:777–8.

71. Wu Y, Wang J, Scott PG, et al. Bone marrow-derived stem cells in wound healing: a review. Wound Repair Regen 2007;1(Suppl 15):S18–26.

72. Metcalfe AD, Ferguson MW. Tissue engineering of replacement skin: the crossroads of biomaterials, wound healing, embryonic development, stem cells and regeneration. J R Soc Interface 2007;4:413–37.

73. MacNeil S. Progress and opportunities for tissue-engineered skin. Nature 2007;445:874–80.

Skin Tissue Engineering—In Vivo and In Vitro Applications

Florian Groeber[a,b,1], Monika Holeiter[a,c,1],
Martina Hampel[a,b], Svenja Hinderer[a,c],
Katja Schenke-Layland[a,c,*]

KEYWORDS

- Tissue engineering • Extracellular matrix • Skin
- In vitro models • Keratinocytes • Melanocytes

INTRODUCTION

The skin is the largest organ in mammals and serves as a protective barrier at the interface between the human body and the surrounding environment. It guards the underlying organs and protects the body against pathogens and microorganisms. Accordingly, it is directly exposed to potentially harmful microbial, thermal, mechanical and chemical influences. In the past 25 years, great efforts have been made to create substitutes that mimic human skin.[1] These skin substitutes were made possible by employing advanced tissue engineering (TE) approaches and have been used for clinical applications, promoting the healing of acute and chronic wounds, or utilized as complex human-based organ-like test systems for basic or pharmaceutical research.[2] In skin TE, various biological and synthetic materials are combined with in vitro-cultured cells to generate functional tissues (**Fig. 1**).[3] A critical issue is the ex vivo expansion that is required to obtain sufficient numbers of the needed cells, while preserving the cells' normal phenotype and functionality. Only then these cells can be used for either the generation of skin substitutes that are suitable for transplantation or as in vitro test systems.[4,5] Especially the latter is of growing interest for the field of skin TE.

In this review article, we summarize in vivo and in vitro applications of tissue-engineered skin. We further highlight novel efforts in the design of advanced disease-in-a-dish models for studies ranging from disease etiology to drug development and screening.

IN VIVO APPLICATIONS

There are multiple reasons for skin damage including genetic disorders, acute trauma, chronic wounds or surgical interventions. One of the most common causes for major skin injury is thermal trauma. In the moment the skin is injured, a complex series of events begins: immune cells are attracted to the injury site, new tissue matrix is generated by fibroblasts, followed by keratinocyte re-epithelialization and eventually the revascularization of the wound.[6] This intricate wound healing process is stimulated and controlled by various growth factors and cytokines.[7] However,

This article originally published in *Advanced Drug Delivery Reviews (2011)*, 352–366, Elsevier.

[a] Department of Cell and Tissue Engineering, Fraunhofer-Institute for Interfacial Engineering and Biotechnology (IGB), Nobelstrasse 12, 70569 Stuttgart, Germany
[b] Institute for Interfacial Engineering, Nobelstrasse 12, 70569 Stuttgart, Germany
[c] Faculty of Medicine, Eberhard Karls University Tübingen, Silcherstrasse 7, 72076 Tübingen, Germany
[1] Both authors contributed equally to this manuscript.
* Corresponding author. Department of Cell and Tissue Engineering, Fraunhofer IGB, Nobelstrasse 12, 70569 Stuttgart, Germany.
E-mail address: katja.schenke-layland@igb.fraunhofer.de

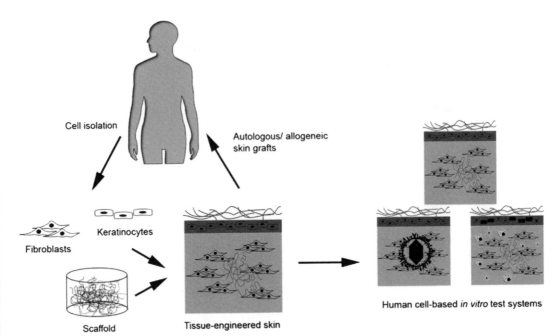

Fig. 1. Schematic illustration of principles of skin tissue engineering. Primary keratinocytes and fibroblasts are isolated from human donor tissues, which are then in vitro expanded prior seeding onto suitable scaffold materials/matrices. For a full-thickness skin equivalent, the fibroblasts and the matrix are initially used to establish the dermal part. The keratinocytes are seeded afterwards on the top of the dermis to ultimately form the epidermal part of the skin substitute. The in vitro-engineered skin can serve as skin graft or can be used as human-cell based in vitro test system.

if the wound healing cascade is negatively affected at any time, healing of the wound might be slowed or the wound can become chronic. When the affected area of skin is too large and therefore cannot be successfully treated with conventional techniques, death of the patient may occur. Skin defects can be divided based on their depth of injury as I) epidermal, II) superficial partial-thickness, III) deep partial-thickness and IV) full-thickness skin wounds.[8] Wounds of the categories I to III can regenerate by the skin's self-healing ability, initiating keratinocyte migration from the wound edges or from hair follicles and sweat glands in the remaining dermis.[9–11] In contrast, the more severe full-thickness skin wounds are specified by a complete destruction of the epithelial regenerative elements that reside in the dermis. Therefore, only epithelialization from the edges of this type of wound is possible. Wound size is a critical factor for epithelialization. Full-thickness wounds with more than 1 cm in diameter need skin grafting to prevent extensive scar formation, resulting in an impaired mobility and cosmetic deformities.[8,12] Due to the use of skin grafts and early excision, a patient with a loss of 50–98% of the total body surface area (TBSA) has a significantly higher survival rate compared with patients

that are treated more conservatively with antimicrobial creams.[13] The perfect graft should be readily available, afflict no immune response, cover and protect the wound bed, enhance the healing process, lessen the pain of the patient and result in little or no scar formation.

Allo- and Autografts

Autologous skin transplantation is currently the clinical gold standard for full-thickness skin wounds including burn injuries.[14,15] Prior to grafting, early excision is an important part of the treatment of burn injuries, as heat-denatured proteins of the skin need to be removed to prevent various complications such as infection, multiple organ dysfunction syndrome, hypertrophic scar formation, uncontrolled inflammatory response or contamination with pathogenic microorganisms.[16] Microorganisms could use the dry scab (eschar) as a source of nutrients and are especially harmful to heavily burnt patients, as this injury also leads to a temporary suppression of cell-mediated and humoral immunity.[17,18] Autologous split skin grafts (SSGs) are harvested with a dermatome that detaches the epidermis and a superficial part of the dermis. Remaining epidermal cells in the residual dermis of the SSG donor site will regrow an epidermis. After application of an SSG to a full-thickness wound, its capillaries merge with the capillary network in the excised wound. This "graft take" is essential for a proper supply of nutrients and ensures graft survival.[15,19] The split skin donor site heals within one week and can be used for SSG harvesting up to 4 times; however, repeated harvesting is associated with scarring at the donor sites as well as lengthy hospital stays. Moreover, in the case of a more extensive injury, donor sites are extremely limited and might leave the patient with too little undamaged skin to harvest enough autologous SSGs. While in 1952 only half of all pediatric burn patients with 50% TBSA burns survived, to date, most children recover from such an injury. Additionally, current data shows a 50% survival rate for children with extensive (98% TBSA) burns.[20] This significant decline in burn mortality is apart from the use of autografts due to other techniques such as early excision, improved fluid resuscitation and infection control.[13,20,21] An early and permanent wound closure is desirable, as it results in minimal or no scarring complications, lower mortality and better functional long-term results.[22] In contrast, wound closure delay is directly proportional to severe hypertrophic scarring. To address the problem of limited SSG harvesting sites, a meshing technique is used that stretches the graft and therefore can cover a larger wounded area at the expense of cosmetic and functional outcome.[12]

Another possibility is the use of allografts (cadaveric skin), for a temporary prevention of fluid loss or contamination of the wound.[23] These allografts can be obtained for example from non-profit European skin banks; however, there is not enough tissue available to meet the current demand and only a few of these tissue banks exist worldwide. Allografts incorporate into deep wounds and provide pain relief; however, ethical as well as safety issues remain, as the rigorous screening for viral diseases and standardized sterilization techniques cannot completely eliminate the possibility of infective agent transmission.[12] In comparison to autologous SSGs, a major disadvantage of allografts is that they leave the patients for weeks with wounds prone to complications. Eventually, allografts undergo immunogenic rejection and the site of injury needs to be covered with an autologous SSG.[24] Delayed rejection can occur in patients with extensive burns due to their pathologically suppressed immune response, but eventually can be triggered by the highly immunogenic epithelial cells of the allograft during its vascularization. Accordingly, there is a great need for an alternative that can provide a more permanent solution.

Tissue-engineered Skin Substitutes

Bioengineered cell-free as well as allogeneic cell-containing skin substitutes provide a possible off-the-shelve solution to the problem of donor graft shortage. These bioengineered skin substitutes offer protection from fluid loss and contamination, while also delivering dermal matrix components, cytokines, and growth factors to the wound bed, enhancing natural host wound healing responses. Bioengineered skin substitutes can be used as temporary coverings after wound debridement until there is an autograft available. After incorporation, these structures persist in the wound during healing or even thereafter. Cell-free biomaterial-based skin substitutes can be used in combination with autografts (whole grafts as well as meshed grafts) as a protective covering over meshed autografts[25,26] and to support their take[27] as well as to stimulate the wound bed in the interstices or to improve graft engraftment in areas of mechanical stress (joints and arm pit).[28] However, in contrast to autografts, tissue-engineered allogeneic skin grafts might bear the risk of transmitting viruses such as hepatitis B Virus (HBV) or Human Immunodeficiency Virus (HIV). One advantage over autologous in vitro-engineered skin substitutes is that they have reduced manufacturing costs.

Epidermal substitutes

For the production of epidermal substitutes, a skin biopsy of 2–5 cm^2 must be taken from the patient. This can be combined with the initial debridement of the burn patient. Subsequently, the epidermis is separated from the dermis and single keratinocytes are enzymatically released and cultured on mitotically inactivated mouse fibroblasts. The used expansion medium contains fetal calf serum and other necessary supplements; however, it is also possible to expand these cells in xenogeneic-free conditions. Currently commercially available autologous epidermal substitutes for clinical use are listed in **Table 1**. There have been several studies testing epithelial allografts like Celaderm[29–31]; however, the effectiveness and safety of these products must be confirmed in controlled clinical studies. In addition to these customized constructs, there have been many groups producing cultured epithelial allografts.[31–35] Allogeneic products have the advantage of reduced manufacturing costs compared to autologous products. Nevertheless, a shortcoming of both products is that they show poor attachment rates that can lead to the formation of blisters.[36]

Dermal substitutes

For the treatment of full-thickness burns, both the epidermal and the dermal layers of the skin need

Table 1
Commercially available epidermal constructs for clinical use

Brand Name/Manufacturer	Graft Type			Cell Source	Biomaterial	Life-span
	Cell-free	Cell-based	Cell-seeded Scaffold (TE)			
CellSpray Clinical Cell Culture (C3), Perth, Australia		x		Autologous keratinocytes	—	Permanent
Epicel Genzyme Biosurgery, Cambridge, MA, USA		x, cell sheet		Autologous keratinocytes	—	Permanent
EpiDex Modex Therapeutiques, Lausanne, Switzerland		x, cell sheet		Autologous keratinocytes	—	Permanent
EPIBASE Laboratoires Genevrier, Sophia-Antipolis, Nice, France		x, cell sheet		Autologous keratinocytes	—	Permanent
MySkin CellTran Ltd, Sheffield, UK			x	Autologous keratinocytes	Synthetic, silicone support layer with a specially formulated surface coating	Permanent
Laserskin or Vivoderm Fidia Advanced Biopolymers, Padua, Italy			x	Autologous keratinocytes	Recombinant, (HAM)	Permanent
Bioseed-S BioTissue TechnologiesGmbH, Freiburg, Germany			x	Autologous keratinocytes	Allogeneic, fibrin sealant	Permanent

Abbreviation: HAM, hyaluronic acid membrane (microperforated).

to be replaced, as the treatment with cultured epidermal (keratinocyte) sheets alone would result in an inferior outcome. In contrast to cultured epidermal sheets, engineered dermal constructs can prevent wound contraction and they provide a greater mechanical stability. The dermal and epidermal equivalents must be applied consecutively, as good dermal vascularization by the debrided wound bed needs to be achieved prior to application of the epidermal layer.[13] There are a wide variety of marketed dermal constructs; both natural and synthetic (**Table 2**). Some of these substitutes are chemically treated allografts (eg, Alloderm(r)), lacking the cellular elements that are responsible for the immunogenic rejection.[37] In contrast, Dermagraft(r) consists of human foreskin fibroblasts, cultured in a biodegradable polyglactin mesh.[38,39] In these substitutes, cells secrete extracellular matrix (ECM) proteins, a variety of growth factors and cytokines into the wound until they undergo normal apoptosis a few weeks post-implantation.

Epidermal/dermal substitutes

The most advanced and sophisticated constructs that are available for clinical use are substitutes that mimic both epidermal as well as dermal layers of the skin. Currently available epidermal/dermal substitutes that are in clinical use are listed in **Table 3**. These constructs are composed of autologous and allogeneic skin cells (keratinocytes and fibroblasts), which are incorporated into scaffolds.[12] Although mimicking the histoarchitecture of normal skin, the epidermal/dermal skin substitutes should be considered as temporary biologically active wound dressings.[38] Skin substitutes provide growth factors, cytokines and ECM for host cells, initiate/regulate wound healing and can result in effective pain relief. Major pitfalls are the high manufacturing costs and their failure to close the wound permanently due to tissue rejection. The immunogenic tolerance of a host towards allogeneic fibroblasts is controversially discussed. There are many reports supporting the hypotheses that allogeneic fibroblasts are tolerated by the host. Therefore, a long-term grafting of these cells up to two months is possible.[41–48] Still, these findings could not be supported by some clinical studies, testing the performance of allogeneic fibroblasts that have been transplanted onto burn wounds.[39] While the use of allogeneic fibroblasts might be sufficient, allogeneic keratinocytes are usually rejected by the host,[40,41] therefore only autologous keratinocytes are adequate for the generation of a permanent epidermal/dermal skin substitute. TissueTech Autograft System designed by Fidia Advanced

Biopolymers is currently the only commercially available product that allows permanent wound closure. It is based on autologous fibroblasts and keratinocytes, grown on microperforated hyaluronic acid membranes[42–44] and is comprised of Hyalograft(r) as a dermal substitute and Laserskin as the epidermal substitute.[45] Because it combines these two independent biomaterials, which need to be applied consecutively to the wound, it cannot be considered a 'true' dermal-epidermal skin substitute. A promising new construct that is not yet commercially available is the Cincinnati Shriners Skin Substitute or Perma-Derm™. This three-dimensionally (3D) reconstructed skin graft, which was designed by Boyce and colleagues,[40,56] is based on a collagen sponge that is seeded with autologous fibroblasts and keratinocytes. It provides permanent wound closure and can be described as a true dermal-epidermal skin substitute.

Despite all efforts, an off-the-shelf, full-thickness skin replacement is not yet available. A future prospective is to incorporate cellular growth-enhancing substances or additional cell types, besides keratinocytes and fibroblasts, in the bio-engineered skin substitutes to obtain constructs with improved function and higher resemblance to native skin. Since poor vascularization of skin grafts is still an unsolved problem, many attempts have been made to improve the angiogenesis in transplanted grafts. A common approach is to stimulate the formation of a capillary network by applying growth factors such as vascular endothelial growth factor (VEGF)[46]; however, these approaches were not successful, because the lifespan of VEGF in the tissue[47] and the blood stream[48] is extremely short. An improved approach is to use drug delivery systems in which growth factors, cDNA or growth factor-producing genetic modified cells are inoculated.[49] Accordingly, a time-dependent release of growth factors is possible. Apart from the stimulation of angiogenesis, endothelial cells (ECs) can be integrated directly into the graft, which leads to a faster formation of capillary like structures in skin substitutes grafted on to mice.[50] Furthermore, melanocytes may be incorporated to obtain a uniform pigmentation[51] and therefore achieve protection from ultra violet (UV) irradiation.[52,53] The addition of skin appendages like hair follicles, sweat glands and sebaceous glands would further improve appearance as well as skin function and wound healing quality of severe burn patients.

Since more than 20 years, hair follicles have been cultured in collagen matrices,[54,55] or they have been maintained free-floating in supplemented Williams E medium.[56] These methods

Table 2
Commercially available dermal constructs for clinical use

| Brand Name/Manufacturer | Graft Type | | | Cell Source | Biomaterial | Life-span |
	Cell-free	Cell-based	Cell-seeded Scaffold (TE)			
AlloDerm LifeCell Corporation, Branchburg, NJ, USA	x			—	Allogeneic human acellular lyophilized dermis	Permanent
Karoderm Karocell Tissue Engineering AB, Karolinska University Hospital, Stockholm, Sweden	x			—	Allogeneic human acellular dermis	Permanent
SureDerm HANS BIOMED Corporation, Seoul, Korea	x			—	Allogeneic human acellular lyophilized dermis	Permanent
GraftJacket Wright Medical Technology, Inc., Arlington, TN, USA	x			—	Allogeneic human acellular pre-meshed dermis	Permanent
Matriderm Dr Suwelack Skin and HealthCare AG, Billerbeck, Germany	x			—	Xenogeneic bovine non-cross-linked lyophilized dermis, coated with α-elastin hydrolysate	Permanent
Permacol Surgical Implant Tissue Science Laboratories plc, Aldershot, UK	x			—	Xenogeneic porcine acellular diisocyanite cross-linked dermis	Permanent
OASIS Wound Matrix Cook Biotech Inc, West Lafayette, IN, USA	x			—	Xenogeneic porcine acellular lyophilized small intestine submucosa	Permanent
EZ Derm Brennen Medical, Inc., MN, USA	x			—	Xenogeneic porcine aldehyde cross-linked reconstituted dermal collagen	Temporary

Product		Cells	Composition	Duration
Integra Dermal Regeneration Template Integra NeuroSciences, Plainsboro, NJ, USA	x	—	Xenogeneic and synthetic: polysiloxane, bovine cross-linked reconstituted	Semi-permanent
Terudermis Olympus Terumo Biomaterial Corp., Tokyo, Japan	x	—	Xenogeneic and synthetic: silicone, bovine lyophilized cross-linked collagen sponge made of heat-denatured collagen	Semi-permanent
Pelnac Standard/Pelnac Fortified Gunze Ltd, Medical Materials Center, Kyoto, Japan	x	—	Xenogeneic and synthetic: silicone/silicone fortified with silicone gauze TREX, atelocollagen derived from pig tendon	Semi-permanent
Biobrane/Biobrane-L UDL Laboratories, Inc., Rockford, IL, USA	x	—	Xenogeneic and synthetic: silicone film, nylon fabric, porcine collagen	Temporary
Hyalomatrix PA Fidia Advanced Biopolymers, Abano Terme, Italy	x	—	Allogeneic and synthetic: HYAFF layered on silicone membrane	Semi-permanent
TransCyte (DermagraftTC) Advanced BioHealing, Inc., New York, NY and La Jolla, CA, USA		Neonatal allogeneic fibroblasts (x)	Xenogeneic and synthetic: silicone film, nylon mesh, porcine dermal collagen	Temporary
Dermagraft Advanced BioHealing, Inc., New York, NY and La Jolla, CA, USA		Neonatal allogeneic fibroblasts (x)	Allogeneic and synthetic: PGA/PLA, ECM	Temporary
Hyalograft 3D Fidia Advanced Biopolymers, Abano Terme, Italy		Autologous fibroblasts (x)	Allogeneic: HAM	Permanent

Abbreviations: ECM, extracellular matrix; HAM: hyaluronic acid membrane (microperforated); PGA: polyglycolic acid (Dexon); PLA: polylactic acid (Vicryl).

Table 3
Commercially available epidermal/dermal constructs for clinical use

Brand Name/ Manufacturer	Graft Type			Cell Source	Biomaterial	Life-span
	Cell-free	Cell-based	Cell-seeded Scaffold (TE)			
Apligraf Organogenesis Inc., Canton, Massachusetts, CA, USA			x	Allogeneic keratinocytes and fibroblasts	Bovine collagen	Temporary
OrCel Ortec International, Inc., New York, NY, USA			x	Allogeneic keratinocytes and fibroblasts	Bovine collagen sponge	Temporary
PolyActive HC Implants BV, Leiden, The Netherlands			x	Autologous keratinocytes and fibroblasts	Synthetic, ... (PEO/PBT)	Temporary
TissueTech Autograft System (Laserskin and Hyalograft 3D) Fidia Advanced Biopolymers, Abano Terme, Italy			x	Autologous keratinocytes and fibroblasts	Recombinant, HAM	Temporary

Abbreviations: HAM, hyaluronic acid membrane (microperforated); PBT, polybutylene terephthalate; PEO, polyethylene oxide terephthalate.

allow the analysis of the development and growth of hair follicles obtained from hairy skin, for example by collagenase digestion of dermis or by microdissection. The integration however of skin appendages (eg, hair) into a graft for the treatment of patients with severe burns still represents a major challenge. In an attempt to address this issue, a recent study tested whether sweat glands could be integrated into engineered skin constructs.[61] Sweat gland cells (SGCs) were cultured on EGF-containing gelatin microspheres, which formed SGC-microsphere complexes. Upon culture of these complexes on engineered skin constructs, sweat gland-like structures developed in vitro. Another study employed porcine embryonic skin precursors (PESPs), isolated from black and haired Guizhou mini pig embryos, that generated epidermis, dermis, rete ridges and appendages, including hair follicles and black hair, sweat glands and sebaceous glands.[57] A suspension of PESPs was applied to the wound of a nude mouse. The wound was protected by adult white Bama mini pig skin pieces. After 4 weeks of implantation, black-pigmented skin and hair became visible. Histology of the growing embryonic skin implants showed that the cambiums from E56 PESP implants contained epidermis and dermis with apparent dermal papillae and rete ridges as well as hair follicles, sebaceous glands and sweat gland ducts. The authors observed no teratoma formation after transplantation of PESPs in the gestational age E56 or later. Although this study provides new hope for the reconstruction of extensive burns, it must be shown that similar success can be achieved using a clinically relevant cell source and an appropriate animal model. However, the hypothesis to advance current skin grafting technologies using autologous derivable stem or progenitor cells[58–60] that possess the potential to generate skin and its appendages might be a promising approach in order to regenerate injured skin.

IN VITRO APPLICATIONS

Tissue-engineered human skin has been developed to reproduce key structural and functional aspects of natural skin. Besides their use as in vivo grafts, as was described above, recently, other applications have emerged for skin substitutes as in vitro test systems[2] (**Fig. 1**). In this context, they enable not only the investigation of fundamental processes in the skin, but also the hazard assessment of various chemical compounds that are topically applied on the skin without the need to use animal models. Results gained from experiments conducted in animal models are often of limited value due to differences in the metabolism and the anatomical architecture compared to human skin (**Fig. 2**). Accordingly, the human identity of skin grafted on an athymic mouse is easily revealed by simple histological staining.[62] In vitro experiments in two-dimensional (2D) monolayer cultures of human cells are also of low relevance due to the lack of complex cell-cell and cell-ECM interactions.[63] However, tissue-engineered skin substitutes can overcome these problems by using human-derived cells that are arranged in a 3D physiological environment, allowing the interaction of the different cell types with one another and the surrounding matrix. Currently, skin substitutes are used in pharmacological research and in basic research. In pharmacological studies, skin substitutes serve as reliable model systems to identify irritative, toxic or corrosive properties of chemical agents that come into contact with the human skin.[64] In basic research, skin substitutes can help to elucidate fundamental processes in the skin such as the stimuli that lead to the formation of the epidermis,[65,66] the molecular cross-talk between different cell types,[67,68] the maintenance of the stem cells,[67] the process of wound healing,[69] and the infection with different kinds of pathogens.[71,72] One great advantage of skin substitutes is that the cellular composition is completely controllable by the researcher. Thus, a certain cell type can be specifically integrated

or omitted to determine the relevance of the cell type in the biological process under investigation. To date, many types of skin substitutes have been developed by different groups.[67,69,70,72–76] Some of these are commercially available such as Skinethic™ RHE, Episkin™ (SkinEthic/L'Oreal, France), Epiderm™, Epiderm FT™ (MatTek Corporation, USA), EST1000, and AST2000 (CellSytems, Germany) (**Table 4**). These skin substitutes can be classified in two types. The first type consists of keratinocytes seeded on a synthetic or collagen carrier simulating only the human epidermis (epidermal substitutes). The second type consists additionally of a dermal layer of human fibroblasts embedded in various kinds of scaffolds (full-thickness skin substitutes) (**Fig. 3**). Possible applications for epidermal and full-thickness skin substitutes as in vitro test systems will be reviewed in the following section.

In Vitro Models

The human skin is exposed to a great amount of different chemicals that need to be classified according to their capacity to harm the skin. The process is defined as corrosive if the skin is irreversibly damaged,[70] whereas the process is defined as irritative, if the skin is reversibly altered.[71] To analyze the possibility of chemicals to harm tissue, Drazie and colleagues in 1944 developed an assay that is based on the topical application of test substances to albino rabbit skin for periods from 4 h to 48 h.[72] With some modifications this assay is still in use; however, apart from being ethically questionable, tests based on the Drazie assay tend to give inaccurate information.[73,74] Hence, current policies are moving towards the use of alternative in vitro test systems. In the EU, the 7th amendment of the

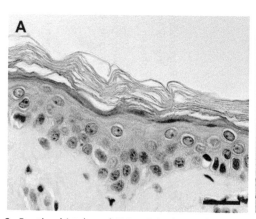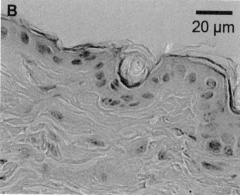

Fig. 2. Routine histology (H&E staining) reveals significant anatomical and morphological differences between human (A) and mouse (B) skin. Scale bars equal 20 μm.

Table 4
Commercially available in vitro epidermal and full-thickness skin substitutes

Brand Name/ Manufacturer	Scaffold Material	Cell Source	Dermis	Test Method	OECD Test Guideline
Episkin™/L'Oreal Nice, France	Collagen	Keratinocytes (mammary/abdominal samples obtained from healthy consenting donors during plastic surgery)	No	Skin irritation Skin corrosion	(No. to be determined) TG 431
Skinethic™ RHE/L'Oreal, Nice, France	Polycarbonate membrane	Keratinocytes (neonatal foreskin tissue or adult breast tissue)	No	Skin irritation Skin corrosion	(No. to be determined) TG 431
Epiderm™/MatTek Corporation, Ashland MA, USA	Collagen-coated, polycarbonate membrane	Human keratinocytes (neonatal foreskin, adult breast skin)	No	Skin irritation Skin corrosion	(No. to be determined) TG 431
EpiDermFT™/MatTek Corporation, Ashland MA, USA	Collagen	Human keratinocytes (neonatal foreskin, adult breast skin), human fibroblasts (neonatal skin, adult skin)	Yes	(No. to be determined)	(No. to be determined)
EST-1000/CellSystems, Troisdorf, Germany	Polycarbonate membrane	Keratinocytes (neonatal foreskin)	No	Skin corrosion	TG 431
AST-2000/CellSystems, Troisdorf, Germany	Collagen	Human keratinocytes Human fibroblasts	Yes	(No. to be determined)	(No. to be determined)
Phenion(r) FT Model/ Henkel AG&Co.KGaA Duesseldorf, Germany	Bovine, cross linked, lyophilized collagen	Primary human keratinocytes (neonatal foreskin), human fibroblasts (neonatal foreskin)	Yes	(No. to be determined)	(No. to be determined)
StrataTest(r)/Stratatech Corporation Madison WI, USA	Collagen I	immortalized, human NIKS(r) keratinocytes dermal fibroblasts	Yes	(No. to be determined)	(No. to be determined)

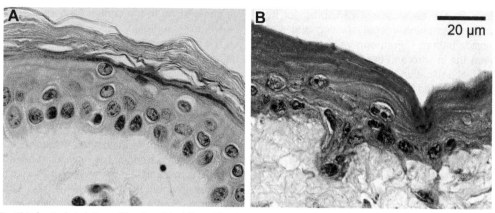

Fig. 3. Histological staining of in vivo skin (*A*) and in vitro-engineered epidermal/dermal skin substitute (*B*). Scale bar equals 20 μm.

"Cosmetics Directive" stated that all animal experiments concerning cutaneous resorption must be replaced by alternative in vitro tests by the year 2009.[75] In this context, the 3R-principles "replace, reduce and refine" were introduced. These principles state that tests should be refined by minimizing the stress for animals by adequate housing, health care and the use of narcosis (Refine), the number of animals that are tested should be reduced (Reduce) and tests should be replaced by in vitro methods (Replace).[76] In contrast, increasingly more substances require testing for possible harmful side effects, as stated by the new European Community regulation on chemicals and their safe use.[77] Therefore the European program for the Registration, Evaluation, Authorization and Restriction of Chemicals (REACH) was introduced with the aim to improve the protection of human health and the environment through the better and earlier identification of the intrinsic properties of chemical substances.[78] Utilizing conventional test methods, the necessary number of toxicity tests will be extremely time and cost consuming. In contrast, skin in vitro models offer a viable and cost-effective alternative for the hazard assessments of the substances under REACH regulatory.

The first in vitro tests were developed to distinguish between corrosive and non-corrosive substances. One approach was to measure the change of the Transcutaneous Electrical Resistances (TER) of human or rabbit skin patches, caused by the application of corrosive agents (TER Method).[79] In the Corrositex™ approach a macromolecular membrane of proteins is used to simulate the barrier function of the skin.[80,81] Corrosive substances are able to destroy the membrane and lead to a color shift in an underlying chemical detection liquid. Furthermore, assays

were developed that are based on tissue-engineered living skin substitutes.[82] To determine the corrosive capacities of test substances, usually 5-dimethylthiazol-2-yl-2,5-diphenyltetrazolium bromide (MTT) assays, together with histological hematoxylin and eosin staining were used. These assays have the advantage of greater availability and better resemblance of human in vivo skin. To determine if these tests can be converted into standardized assays that are able to replace the Drazie test, they were evaluated together with two methods based on living skin substitutes (Episkin™ and Skin²™) by the European Center for the Validation of Alternative Methods (ECVAM). This validation study showed that the Episkin™ model can reliably distinguish between corrosive and non-corrosive substances and is therefore able to replace animal experiments.[83] Since then, more corrosion assays based on skin substitutes have been developed[84,85] and the EpiDerm™, the SkinEthic™ and the EST-1000 method were validated according to ECVAM regulatory for corrosion testing.[86–88] Unlike the assays for acute corrosion, skin irritation tests are more complex and need not only the measurement of cytotoxicity, but also of metabolic reactions such as cytokines and enzyme release.[71] In response to physical or chemical stresses, keratinocytes release various substances such as interleukin-1α (IL-1 α), interleukin-8 (IL-8), tumor necrosis factor α (TNF-α), interleukin-6 (IL-6), interleukin-7 (IL-7), and interleukin-15 (IL-15) in vivo.[71] Employing in vitro skin substitutes, a dose-dependent release of the cytosolic enzyme lactate dehydrogenase (LDH) and IL-1α was observed in response to the application of various cosmetics.[89] Another assay based on the measurement of IL-1α, IL-8 and MTT was able to classify a broad variety of test substances according to their irritation potential.[90] This was followed by the development of a protocol that uses only membrane integrity testing and IL-1α expression pattern.[85] Furthermore, the correlation between the in vitro and in vivo data determined irritation classification of 22 cosmetic products was demonstrated[99] leading to the validation of the EpiSkin™, Epiderm SIT™ and SkinEthic™ RHE assay according to ECVAM guidelines.[91–94] Due to the development and validation of the described in vitro corrosion and irritation tests, the number of necessary animal experiments could already be reduced significantly. However, skin substitutes cannot be used to replace all animal experiments because no systemic response of an applied substance can be investigated thus far.

Currently, many drugs and cosmetics are applied to the skin, but the amount of the substances that reach the targeted site remains often unclear. Hence, for the cosmetic industry, it is of great interest to have an in vitro system, which can determine how much of a cosmetic formula penetrates through the epidermal layer into the skin.[95] Furthermore, it is crucial to analyze where a substance has an effect, either locally in the skin or systemically through the distribution in the vascular system (transdermal delivery).[96] Penetration assays can thereby help to determine the risk/benefit ratio of certain chemicals such as glucocorticoids.[97] Currently, researchers are investigating the penetration of substances through artificial stratum corneum (SC),[96] epidermal reconstructs[95] and epidermal/dermal[98] reconstructs. A great advantage of these artificial models is not only that the healthy state of the skin can be mimicked, but also that it is possible to simulate diseased states.[99] However, a major difference between in-vivo skin and skin substitutes is the presence of skin appendages such as hair follicles, sweat glands and sebaceous glands. These appendages represent openings, which can increase the permeability of the skin. Percutaneous absorption of drugs is due to two different routes of passive diffusion. The transepidermal diffusion uses an inter- or transcellular pathway across the stratum corneum, whereas the transappendageal diffusion follows the route through the hair follicles and their associated sebaceous glands.[100] The importance of skin appendages and their ability to act as a conduit for drug transport have been recognized[101,102] and could be confirmed by experiments on a tissue-engineered human skin equivalent with hair.[103] This model was designed from human fibroblasts and keratinocytes in which complete pilosebaceous units, obtained by thermolysin digestion of hairy skin, were inserted. In a hydrocortisone diffusion test, this model could show a significantly increased rate of penetration in comparison to the control (skin equivalent with sham hair insertion).

The skin is exposed to potentially harmful irradiation that can cause serious alterations in the skin. To protect the exposed cells, the natural skin is pigmented with melanin that is able to absorb harmful UV radiation (UVA and UVB) and can scavenge formed radical oxygen species.[104] Melanin itself is produced in melanocytes and distributed to the surrounding keratinocytes through dendritic extensions.[105] Hence, the investigation of skin reactions to sunlight requires the addition of melanocytes in order to mimic the in vivo situation correctly. By introducing melanocytes into skin substitutes, the natural process of pigmentation could be successfully recreated in vitro.[106–108] Furthermore, in these models the effects of UVB radiation were investigated at the cellular level.[109] By using cells from different donors with a high phototype (dark hair/dark skin) and low phototype (fair hair/pale skin), it was even possible to simulate different phototypes in vitro. Such models were used to investigate the impaired photo protective properties of skin from individuals with a low phototype.[110] In another approach, chimeric skin substitutes were generated that contained different combinations of keratinocytes and melanocytes from Caucasian and Negroid donors. Using these chimeric skin substitutes, it could be demonstrated that the pigmentation is under the control of the melanocytes, whereas the keratinocytes contribute to the photo protection, due to their antioxidant defense system. The exposure of the skin to sunlight can lead to erythema and even the development of live threatening melanoma.[111] To protect natural skin in vivo from damaging radiation, sun-blocking lotions can be applied topically. To develop improved photo protective agents, skin substitutes can be used as easy manageable in vitro test systems.[112] The combination of systemically or topically applied drugs together with sun irradiation can also result in adverse skin reaction. This phototoxicity can result in amplified erythema and inflammatory responses in vivo. To predict the phototoxic effects of substances, skin substitutes can be exposed to drugs and UVB irradiation in vitro. It has been demonstrated that epidermal skin substitutes are able to discriminate between phototoxic and non-phototoxic substances and are thus a suitable alternative test method for phototoxicity.[113]

Full-thickness in Vitro Models

Although the great majority of the skin substitutes used in pharmacological research are only composed of an epidermal layer, these skin substitutes could be further improved by the addition of a dermal layer containing fibroblasts. In this context, fibroblasts have only recently begun to receive more attention. It was discovered that skin fibroblasts are far from being homogeneous and it was speculated that some chronic wounds are due to a change in the composition of the fibroblast population.[114] Using standard cell culture, it was shown that fibroblasts positively influence keratinocyte growth in vitro, most likely due to the fact that these cells secrete soluble growth factors.[115] In natural skin, the interaction between fibroblasts and keratinocytes plays a major role in processes such as wound healing[116] and the formation of the base membrane.[117,118] Using skin substitutes, it was demonstrated that fibroblasts play a crucial role in the natural epidermal histogenesis. Without fibroblasts, the keratinocyte differentiation is severely affected and results only in few layers of highly differentiated epithelial cells.[67,68] Interestingly, keratinocytes have also a positive effect on the proliferation of fibroblasts.[67] This interaction of epidermal and dermal cells is hypothesized to be due to a double-paracrine mechanism that regulates the growth of keratinocytes and fibroblasts.[119,120] According to this hypothesis, keratinocytes secrete IL-1 that stimulates the skin fibroblasts to secret keratinocyte growth factor (KGF) and granulocyte-monocyte colony-stimulating factor (GM-CSF), which in turn positively influence the proliferation of the keratinocytes. Furthermore, dermal fibroblasts play an essential role in the remodeling of the skin, in the contraction of acute wounds[121,122] and they can increase the resistances of keratinocytes to toxic chemicals.[123] Based on these findings, one could conclude that in order to gain meaningful data from toxicological in vitro studies, the isolated focus on a keratinocyte-containing epidermal layer alone is not sufficient, making the use of a full-thickness skin model essential. In contrast, epidermal substitutes might be more suitable for the determination of the penetration coefficient through the skin. In routine in vitro penetration studies (= percutaneous absorption testing), a defined area of a skin substitute separates a donor from an acceptor chamber. The leak-proof connection of the skin substitute to the experimental setup is important. Collagen-based full-thickness skin substitutes are not ideal for such tests since they do not seal the whole surface area due to a low mechanic resilience, thus resulting in open edges, through which the substance under investigation can openly diffuse.[98]

Bell et al. described the first process for generating an in vitro test system with a dermal and an epidermal component.[122] In this process, allogeneic fibroblasts were seeded into a matrix of bovine collagen type I. In order to generate a natural epidermis, keratinocytes were cultured on the surface of this matrix at an air-liquid interface.[124] This skin substitute has been used under the name Apligraf™ for the treatment of chronic wounds and was marketed under the name TESTSKIN™ as an in vitro test system.[125] To date, different techniques for the formation of a dermal layer ex vivo have been described. Fibroblasts are seeded into a hydrated gel of collagen,[126] a fibrin gel[127] or a scaffold composed of collagen/chitosan/chondroitin-4-6-sulfates.[128] Furthermore, the use of small intestine submucosa (SIS) has been described.[129] In another approach, high densities of fibroblasts were seeded onto a synthetic membrane. Over time, the fibroblasts generated their own matrix, which could then be inoculated with keratinocytes to form a skin substitute (self assembly method).[74,75] The advantage of this method is that no cross-species scaffold is needed for the formation of a dermal layer. Furthermore, synthetic polymers such as polylactic-co-glycolic acid (PLGA),[130] polycaprolactone (PCL),[131] a combination of PLGA/PCL[132] or PLGA and PCL with naturally derived collagen[105,133] were used to generate the dermal skin layer. The advantages of these polymers include a greater mechanic stability and no risk of pathogen transfer. However, major pitfalls of these materials are a lack of natural adhesion and signaling molecules.

Full-thickness skin substitutes are of great value for the investigation of complex dermatological questions, where the molecular crosstalk between the keratinocytes and the fibroblasts is crucial. Furthermore, full-thickness skin substitutes are necessary for the investigation of processes where the epidermis and the dermis are equally involved. In order to test possible immunological reactions on skin, Langerhans cells (LCs) can be introduced into full-thickness skin substitutes. The function of these specialized dendritic cells (DCs) of the skin is to capture and process antigens that come into contact with the skin. LCs reside as immature cells in epidermal niches.[134] Upon binding to an antigen, these cells migrate from the epidermis into local dermal lymph nodes. During this migration, the LCs differentiate into mature DCs and can present the processed antigen to T-cells in the lymph nodes.[135] As reported, first attempts of the integration of epidermal LCs into a skin substitute failed and resulted only in round pycnotic cells in the upper layers of the epidermis.[136] However, to overcome these problems, researchers integrated non-differentiated CD34-positive (CD34[+]) hematopoietic progenitor cells (HPCs) and CD34[+] HPCs that were differentiated into LCs by granulocyte macrophage growth factor and tumor necrosis factor-α

(TNF-α), into a pigmented skin substitute.[136] The integration of differentiated as well as non-differentiated cell populations resulted in suprabasally located cells that exhibited LC typical markers. These results provided evidence for the influence of the keratinocytes in the LC differentiation from CD34[+] HPCs.[131,136] In another approach, epidermal biopsies were placed directly onto a dermal substitute of collagen and fibroblasts. The epidermal keratinocytes and the LCs migrated out of the biopsies and covered the dermal compartment. After culture on an air-liquid interface, a functional epidermis was formed that contained LCs with an immature phenotype. To simulate the early contact with an allergen, these skin substitutes were treated with the LCs promoting GM-CSF and the immunosuppressive agent cyclosporine-A (SC-A). GM-CSF was found to increase the migration, but not the density of the LCs, whereas SC-A did not influence the density of immature LCs.[137]

The skin is supplied through a capillary network in the dermis, formed by ECs. As a reaction to the destruction of the capillary network, caused by deep tissue wounds, ECs sprout out of the left capillaries and form new vessels in a process referred as angiogenesis.[137] This process has been extensively investigated in order to improve the neovascularization of transplanted skin grafts. An issue with full-thickness skin grafts is that many of these grafts become necrotic due to an impaired formation of new blood vessels.[138] Many different culture systems were used to investigate angiogenesis.[139–143] These in vitro angiogenesis models are suitable models to study the effect of pro-angiogenic factors,[139,140] anti-angiogenic substances,[138] matrix metalloproteinases (MMPs),[141] cell adhesion molecules[142,143] and fibrolysis.[150,151] Furthermore, ECs were integrated into the dermis of full-thickness skin substitutes.[144–146] These models mimic the in vivo situation more closely and enable the interaction of the ECs with the ECM and the surrounding cells. As a result, ECs formed capillary-like structures in the dermis. However, one reason why no mature blood vessels were produced might be the lack of shear stress for the ECs. In vivo, ECs are exposed to fluid shear stress, induced by the blood flow, that is critical for ECs to exhibit a natural phenotype.[147] But so far no skin substitute with an artificial blood stream has been described, that would allow the culture of ECs under physiological shear conditions.

DISEASE SKIN MODELS

In the skin, the interaction of keratinocytes, fibroblasts, melanocytes and the cells of the immune system is tightly controlled by various factors and cascades. The disruption of this system can result in an uncontrolled proliferation of keratinocytes (as seen in psoriasis) or melanocytes (in malignant melanoma).[148,149] Moreover, the skin is exposed to external influences such as pathogenic microorganisms, viruses and mechanical injuries. The in vitro investigation of these processes in skin substitutes can help to understand the complex processes that underlie these diseases, which is essential for the development of new effective therapies.

Psoriasis Skin Models

Psoriasis is an inflammatory skin disease that results in scaly, reddened skin patches. Hyperproliferation of keratinocytes in affected patches is a common characteristic of psoriasis. Histological staining of biopsies reveals a thickened epidermis that extends deeper into the dermis.[150] In the beginning of the investigation of psoriasis, it was believed that this disease is due to an altered differentiation and proliferation of the keratinocytes.[149] The generation of in vitro skin substitutes using fibroblasts and keratinocytes isolated from patients afflicted by psoriasis helped to gain new insights into this disease. For example, using the TESTSKIN™ model for the investigation of psoriasis, it was demonstrated that fibroblasts from psoriatic donors induce the hyper-proliferation of keratinocytes from healthy donors.[151] It was further found that the origin of the fibroblasts has an impact on the expression of the interferon-γ receptor in the epidermal keratinocytes.[152] In another approach, the induction of psoriatic features in healthy keratinocytes from psoriatic fibroblasts was linked to an increased IL-8 secretion.[153] In addition to these findings, it was discovered that drugs which target cells of the immune system are able to slow the disease.[154] These results were further supported by studies that showed decreasing clinical symptoms through the application of antibodies against CD3/4[155] and an IL-2-diphtheria-toxin fusion protein that targets specifically T-cells.[156] Thus, it is evident that the immune system plays a role in the induction of psoriasis. Recently, new psoriatic skin substitutes were developed and further characterized. One of these systems was based on the self-assembly method.[157] Another one is based on a decellularized dermis.[158] Additionally, researchers were able to induce psoriatic features in skin substitutes from healthy donors through transglutaminase inhibitors[159] and cytokines such as TNF-α, IL-1α, Il-6 and IL-2.[160] Although these models are able to simulate some characteristics of psoriasis in vitro, the contribution of the immune system can still not be analyzed with these skin substitutes. One approach to address this issue is to use psoriatic skin substitutes that are grafted on severe combined immune deficiency mice. In these models, psoriatic phenotypes can be induced by the injection of activated natural killer cells.[161]

In Vitro Melanoma Model

Amongst the disease alterations of the skin, described here, malignant melanoma is the most aggressive and most prominent in the human population. Malignant melanoma develops in a multistep process starting in melanocytes in the epidermis.[148] In this process, melanocytes are located at the base membrane's loose contact to the surrounding keratinocytes and enter a radial growth phase. This radial growth phase is followed by a vertical growth phase in which melanoma cells can penetrate through the base membrane. Genes that are related to this transformation are v-raf murine sarcoma viral oncogene homolog B1 (BRAF), the cyclin-dependent kinase inhibitor 2A (INK4a), microphthalmia-associated transcription factor (MITF), v-kit Hardy-Zuckerman 4 feline

sarcoma viral oncogene homolog (c-KIT), snail homolog 2 (SLUG) and endothelin receptor type B (EDNRB).[162] In addition to this genetic alteration, the disruption of the keratinocyte/melanocyte homeostasis is suggested to be the trigger for the formation of melanoma cells.[163] This hypothesis has been supported by the findings that melanocytes proliferate stronger without the presence of keratinocytes and express melanoma cell adhesion molecule (Mel-CAM/MUC18) receptors that are related to melanoma formation.[164] A reason for the severe progression of the disease is the formation of metastases in different parts of the human body. These metastases are due to a vertical growth phase through the base membrane that separates the dermal from the epidermal layer. The clinical outcome of this invasive behavior is dependent on the molecular interaction of the metastatic cells with the cells of the surrounding tissue. In order to investigate these interactions, 2D cell culture experiments[161,163] or in vivo experiments in different animal models[171,173] were conducted. An alternative to these in vivo tests is to analyze the behavior of melanoma cells in 3D skin substitutes[165] (Fig. 4). These melanoma skin substitutes (MSS)

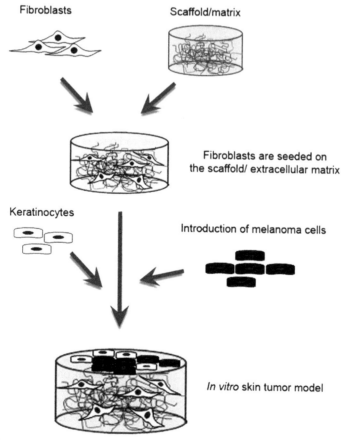

Fig. 4. Schematic of an in vitro-engineered epidermal/dermal skin tumor model with melanoma cells.

can help to close the gap between the two possible model systems by reproducing the 3D arrangement of epidermal and mesenchymal cells in a controlled experimental setup. In different studies, melanoma cells were successfully embedded into skin substitutes.[175,176] These studies investigated the growth behavior of melanoma cell lines associated with cell-cell and cell-matrix interactions. Moreover, the production of growth factors by seeded melanoma cell lines was analyzed. Using these MSS, it was demonstrated that melanoma cell lines from various progression phases behave differently in skin substitutes according to their origin. Melanoma cells from the radial growth phase were not able to cross the base membrane, whereas melanoma cells from the vertical growth phase could penetrate through the base membrane.[166] Furthermore, different cell lines reacted differently to α-Melanocyte stimulating hormone (α-MSH) indicating that melanoma cells with a different genetic background can react differently to therapeutics.[167] It could also be confirmed that the invasive behavior is due to the crosstalk of the melanoma cells with surrounding skin cells.[168] It was further shown that the penetration of melanoma cell lines through the base membrane is dependent on the secretion of metalloproteinase-9 by the keratinocytes.[169] In another experiment, multiphoton laser scanning microscopy was used to investigate the invasive behavior of squamous cell carcinoma (SCC) cells. According to this study, SSC cell invasion is promoted by the aberrant expression of tumor-derived fibronectin in these cells. In great contrast, fibronectin that was derived from normal melanocytes did not contribute to an invasive melanoma cell phenotype.[170]

Skin substitutes can also be used in the development of new anti-melanoma drugs. Due to MSS, the in vitro simulation of the interaction of different drugs or substances with human tissue and melanoma cells has been made possible.[171] This led to the identification of new relevant signaling pathways in the treatment of skin cancer and could potentially help to identify potent new drugs in an early stage of the research. A recent study demonstrated that a combination of the zinc fingers and homeoboxes 2 (RAF) inhibitor sorafenib with the mechanistic target of rapamycin (mTOR) inhibitor rapamycin prevents melanoma cell lines from invading into a dermal skin substitute.[172] Nevertheless, in order to fully investigate tumor angiogenesis and metastasis development in vitro, the vascularization of the currently available MSS will be necessary. In order to outgrow the size of approximately 2–3 mm, tumors need to be supplied with nutrients through the vascular system. Tumors secrete growth factors that attract ECs to form capillaries that supply the melanoma (tumor angiogenesis).[173] Furthermore, melanoma cells can penetrate through the EC layer that is lining the capillary vessels leading to the distribution of melanoma cells throughout the human body that can cause secondary tumors (metastasis).[174] In order to investigate these processes, the development of a vascularized skin substitute is crucial. Such a model could additionally simulate the critical barrier formed by the ECs and would allow the investigation of the molecular signals that are involved in tumor angiogenesis in vitro. Both processes are of great importance, because they can serve as potential targets for new anti-melanoma drugs.

Wound Healing Model

Wound or tissue repair is the result of a series of overlapping events, which can be classified into four phases: hemostasis, inflammation, granulation tissue formation and scar formation. As a result of an injury, platelets aggregate and form a hemostatic plug by converting fibrinogen to fibrin. Besides preventing further loss of blood, platelets release growth factors such as tumor growth factor (TGF-β), platelet derived growth factor (PDGF) as well as several adhesive proteins. These molecules activate cells in the surrounding area. During the inflammatory phase, neutrophils appear at the site of the injury and release a variety of highly active antimicrobial substances like cationic peptides, proteases and reactive oxygen species that are important for wound cleaning and the prevention of infections.[175] Releasing free radicals is another way of wound cleaning; however, these radicals can also harm healthy cells. This situation can particularly be found in chronic wounds.[176] Two days after injury, macrophages arrive at the wound and initiate or engage in multiple processes of functions such as digestion of matrix elements and cell debris,[177] as well as the release of growth factors and cytokines. Moreover, it has been shown that macrophages have the potential to support angiogenesis.[178] In addition, mast cells derived from circulating basophiles and other leukocyte subsets are also considered to be involved in tissue repair by releasing a variety of growth factors and cytokines. Therefore, inflammatory and endothelial cells can enter the site of injury. One part of the granulation tissue formation phase is the re-epithelialization, where keratinocytes migrate into the injured area. Additionally, fibroblasts invade the wound and synthesize new ECM. This granulation tissue consists of glycosaminoglycans, proteoglycans, collagen III, thrombospondin, fibronectin and vitronectin that promote angiogenesis. While massive angiogenic responses take place, the fibroblasts transform into myofibroblasts. These cells bring the margins of the wound together in order to reduce the size of the wound. The last phase of wound healing is the transformation of granulation tissue into scar tissue. Characteristic for the scar formation is a decrease in inflammation and a reduction of capillaries. Myofibroblasts undergo apoptosis and a new collagenous matrix replaces the provisional matrix.[6,176,179] This cascade occurs in normal wound healing, where a reestablishment of the equilibrium between scar formation and scar remodeling takes place. In contrast, the pathological response to an injury may result in fibrosis or chronic ulcers. Fibrosis is characterized by excessive matrix deposition and therefore loss of tissue function.[7] It has been discussed that chronic ulcer formation is depended on the phenotypic differences in fibroblasts at the wound site. The altered fibroblast population is characterized by cells with a low proliferation capacity, a flattened morphology, as well as an increased collagen production that leads to chronic non-healing wounds.[114]

To study the wound healing process in detail, the development of in vitro wound model systems is important. Such in vitro alternatives can easily be manipulated and are cost-effective compared to in vivo systems.[180] There are 3 main approaches: (1) a monolayer cell culture assay, (2) in vitro skin models (**Fig. 5**), and (3) ex vivo skin cultures. One of the simplest wound healing models is the 2D cell monolayer model. Fibroblasts are seeded into culture dishes and are grown to confluence. The monolayer is then wounded by removing a part of the layer with a razor blade.[181] This model is advantageous to study migratory and proliferative responses as well as cytokine release. To investigate protein synthesis, re-epithelialization and proliferation, a more complex model must be used. Native

skin-mimicking in vitro substitutes permit the investigation of responses induced by different stimuli; however, the wound healing process in vivo includes more cell types than only fibroblasts and keratinocytes. Therefore, current efforts are focusing on either the possibility of ex vivo skin long-term cultures[182] or the improvement of skin substitutes.

There are several approaches of inducing a wound including scratching, abrading and burning. The most commonly used instruments to induce injury are mashers, scalpels, biopsy punches, dermatomes, liquid nitrogen and lasers.[69] For the most common injury model - the burn model - the routine approach is using a brass string heat to 150 °C.[183] However, more reproducible wound sizes can be achieved by using a laser. Accordingly, Vaughan et al. showed that they can produce wounds of exactly 6 mm length, 1 mm width and 400 μm depth for determining re-epithelialization and aging in vitro.[184]

In Vitro Infection Models

Candida albicans

C albicans is an asexual ascomycete that can become a serious pathogen for immunosuppressed patients. This fungus is part of the microbial flora of the epidermis and mucous membranes. *C albicans* is a dimorphic fungus that shows inducible alternation between the yeast and hypha form.[185] In order to develop an in vitro model to study the mechanisms of pathogenicity and virulence, commercial available substitutes of the oral[186] and cutaneous[187] epithelium were infected with *C albicans*. The infection of the epidermal substitutes resulted in the typical morphological changes of the epidermis as seen in vivo.[188] Furthermore, the molecular response of the epidermal cells elicited by a *C albicans* infection could be investigated. It could be demonstrated that IL-1α, IL-1β, IL-8, GM-CSF, chemokine (C-C motif) ligand 21C

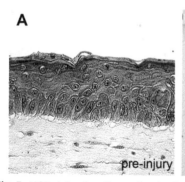
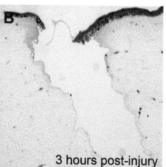
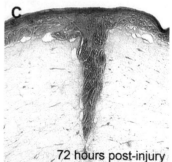

pre-injury   3 hours post-injury   72 hours post-injury

Fig. 5. H&E stained sections of an in vitro human cell-based wound healing model before injury (*A*), as well as 3 h (*B*) and 72 h (*C*) post-injury.

(Exodus-2), TNF-α and P-selectin ligand (PSL) expressions were upregulated; whereas the expression of TNF-β was downregulated.[189] Additionally, epidermal substitutes were used to study the virulence factors that enable *C albicans* to penetrate through the epidermis. In these studies it has been demonstrated that *C albicans* releases a specific pattern of secreted aspartic proteinases (SAPs) during the penetration through the different epidermal layers.[190] The importance of SAPs in the infection process was shown in a further study that demonstrated a significantly reduced capacity of *C albicans* to penetrate through the epidermis, due to the application of SAP inhibitors.[191] To gain new insights into the adhesion and penetration behavior of *C albicans*, our group integrated various *C albicans* mutants into a full-thickness skin substitute.[204] With this new in vitro model we could demonstrate that both morphologies of *C albicans*, yeast as well as hypha, form and adhere to the tissue within 30 min. Furthermore, we were able to monitor the progression of hypha formation as well as the penetration through the epithelium into the dermis. In addition, our group was able to investigate the influence of transcription factors, such as enhanced filamentous growth protein 1 (EFG1) and STE-like transcription factor (CPH1), on the adhesion and invasive behavior of *C albicans*.[204]

Herpes model

3D skin substitutes have been used in the investigation of many viruses including papillomaviruses, adenoviruses, parvoviruses, poxviruses and herpes viruses.[192] The Herpes Simplex Virus (HSV) infection is a common disease of the human skin that results in painful skin lesions. Apart from these local symptoms, HSV can result in acute liver failure[193] or in corneal blindness.[194] HSV is able to infect the epidermal cells leading to the formation of synergic cell clusters and can integrate into the genome of the dorsal root ganglia (DRG) cells, where the virus can stay latent for extended periods of time. During latency only few HSV genes are expressed including the latency associated transcript (LAT). However, the outbreak of HSV infection can be initiated spontaneously or triggered by external stimuli like emotional stress, UV radiation or immunosuppression. If latency is broken, the HSV is axonally transported back to the epidermal layer where it can result in the reappearing of the clinical symptoms.[195]

Skin substitutes have been used to investigate the initial step of HSV infection, in which the virus must penetrate through the epidermis (**Fig. 6**). In these studies, HSV was applied onto full-thickness skin substitutes made out of fibroblasts in a collagen hydrogel with an epidermis comprised of either primary keratinocytes or a keratinocyte cell line. The infection of these skin substitutes resulted in a rapid spreading of the virus in the epidermis and the formation of typical cytopathic effects as seen in vivo.[196,197] To study the protective function of the outermost stratum corneum (SC), skin substitutes were inoculated with HSV before and after the formation of the SC. Typical cytopathic effects in the epidermis were only visible, if HSV was added prior to the formation of the SC. The addition of the HSV after the formation of the SC resulted in no obvious sights of infection. Nevertheless, the expression of HSV LAT genes was detectable, indicating a latent infection of the keratinocyte cell line.[198] Another study investigated the influence of antiviral agents such as acyclovir (ACV), penciclovir (PCV), brivudin (BVDU), foscarnet (PFA), and

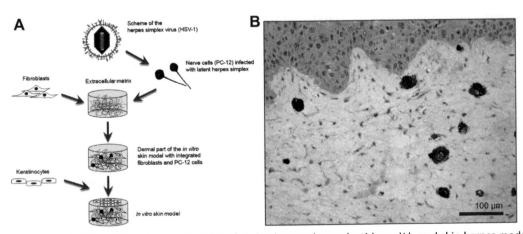

Fig. 6. Schematic (*A*) and (*B*) microscopic views of an in vitro-engineered epidermal/dermal skin herpes model. Scale bar equals 100 μm.

cidofovir (CDV) on the HSV infection using an in vitro model.[199] These studies support that skin substitutes can be used as test systems in the investigation of the infection process of skin cells. However, these models are not suitable for studying the reactivation from the latent state and the following transmission of HSV to the epidermal cells.

The transmission of HSV from the DRG cells to the epidermis was investigated in an in vitro model using a dual chamber with human fetal DRG cells separated from skin explants by an agarose gel. In the experiments, axons grew through the agarose gel into the skin explants, delivering nucleocapsids of the HSV to the epidermal cells.[200] In a follow up study, this transmission was inhibited by poly- and monoclonal antibodies.[200] To study the molecular and cellular mechanisms involved in establishing, maintaining and mediating reactivation from latency, our group recently developed a full-thickness skin substitute in which pheochromocytoma cells (PC12), transfected with the HSV genome, were seeded (see **Fig. 6**B).

CONCLUSIONS

In vitro skin models are currently employed for identifying skin-corrosive or -toxic substances and have been proven to be very useful tools for the investigation of basic developmental processes as well as for the identification of pathological conditions. Although the design of the epidermal and/or dermal layer-mimicking in vitro skin substitutes is today nearly state-of-the-art, there are clearly differences between these models and native in vivo skin.[201] One pitfall of in vitro substitutes is that they are not easily created, prepared or stored. Virtually all in vitro skin is custom-manufactured manually. An automated process would significantly reduce manufacturing costs and would offer the complete control of the process with a reliable outcome. The use of human keratinocyte-derived cell lines that are still able to cornify would help to reduce the price of a skin equivalent even further and improve the predictability of the final construct. Unfortunately, the majority of the currently available cell lines are derived from carcinoma cells, which lack the ability to form a corneous layer; only recently, a new cornifying cell line was introduced.[202] Another factor that is limiting the commercial success of skin substitutes is their short lifespan. It has been reported that skin substitutes manufactured with fibrin as the dermal scaffold material can be cultured up to 12 weeks.[67] One approach to achieve an extended usability is the development of appropriate skin substitute preservation protocols as it had been done for dermal skin grafts.[203]

Future developments in in vitro skin substitutes should include the addition of skin appendages. The integration of sweat glands or hair follicles will help to mimic a more realistic in vivo situation, thus offering a more correct experimental setup. Many advances have been made in the last decades in order to create vascularized full-thickness in vitro skin models; however, the vascular-like structures could not be integrated with an outer vascular system in which physiological shear conditions are sustained, thus the maturation of the in vitro vasculature was prevented. The use of more advanced biological scaffolds or synthetic vasculature-mimicking structures might help to overcome these problems.

ACKNOWLEDGMENTS

The authors kindly thank Shannon Lee Layland and Michaela Kaufmann for their helpful suggestions and comments, Lena Schober (Fraunhofer IGB, Dept. of Cell and Tissue Engineering) for her technical help as well as Ina Hogk (Fraunhofer IGB, Dept. of Molecular Biotechnology) for the histological image of the herpes model. The authors are grateful for the financial support by the Fraunhofer-Gesellschaft Internal Programs (Grant No. Attract 692263 [to K.S.-L.]).

REFERENCES

1. MacNeil S. Progress and opportunities for tissue-engineered skin. Nature 2007;445:874–80.
2. Ponec M. Skin constructs for replacement of skin tissues for in vitro testing. Adv Drug Deliv Rev 2002;54(Suppl 1):S19–30.
3. Vacanti CA, Mikos AG. Tissue Eng 1995;1:1–2.
4. Falkenberg FW, Weichert H, Krane M, et al. In vitro production of monoclonal antibodies in high concentration in a new and easy to handle modular minifermenter. J Immunol Meth 1995;179:13–29.
5. Schade R, Pfister C, Halatsch R, et al. Polyclonal IgY Antibodies from Chicken Egg Yolk-An Alternative to the Production of Mammalian IgG type Antibodies in Rabbits. In: Fund for the Replacement of Animals in Medical Experiments. Nottingham: ATLA; 1991. p. 403–19.
6. Midwood KS, Williams LV, Schwarzbauer JE. Tissue repair and the dynamics of the extracellular matrix. Int J Biochem Cell Biol 2004;36:1031–7.
7. Diegelmann RF, Evans MC. Wound healing: an overview of acute, fibrotic and delayed healing. Front Biosci 2004;9:283–9.
8. Papini R. Management of burn injuries of various depths. BMJ 2004;329:158–60.

9. Blanpain C, Lowry WE, Geoghegan A, et al. Self-renewal, multipotency, and the existence of two cell populations within an epithelial stem cell niche. Cell 2004;118:635–48.

10. Tumbar T. Epithelial skin stem cells. Meth. Enzymol 2006;419:73–99.

11. Tumbar T, Guasch G, Greco V, et al. Defining the epithelial stem cell niche in skin. Science 2004; 303:359–63.

12. Shevchenko RV, James SL, James SE. A review of tissue-engineered skin bioconstructs available for skin reconstruction. J R Soc Interface 2010;7: 229–58.

13. Herndon DN, Barrow RE, Rutan RL, et al. A comparison of conservative versus early excision. Therapies in severely burned patients. Ann Surg 1989;209:547–52 [discussion: 552–543].

14. Stanton RA, Billmire DA. Skin resurfacing for the burned patient. Clin Plast Surg 2002;29:29–51.

15. Andreassi A, Bilenchi R, Biagioli M, et al. Classification and pathophysiology of skin grafts. Clin Dermatol 2005;23:332–7.

16. Zilberman M, Elsner JJ. Antibiotic-eluting medical devices for various applications. J Control Release 2008;130:202–15.

17. Vindenes H, Bjerknes R. Activation of polymorphonuclear neutrophilic granulocytes following burn injury: alteration of Fc-receptor and complement-receptor expression and of opsonophagocytosis. J Trauma 1994;36:161–7.

18. Yamamoto H, Siltharm S, deSerres S, et al. Effect of cyclo-oxygenase inhibition on in vitro B-cell function after burn injury. J Trauma 1996;41:612–9 [discussion: 620-611].

19. Converse JM, Smahel J, Ballantyne DL Jr, et al. Inosculation of vessels of skin graft and host bed: a fortuitous encounter. Br J Plast Surg 1975;28: 274–82.

20. Rose JK, Herndon DN. Advances in the treatment of burn patients. Burns 1997;23(Suppl 1):S19–26.

21. Fratianne RB, Brandt CP. Improved survival of adults with extensive burns. J Burn Care Rehabil 1997;18:347–51.

22. Wolfe RA, Roi LD, Flora JD, et al. Mortality differences and speed of wound closure among specialized burn care facilities. JAMA 1983;250:763–6.

23. Quinby WC Jr, Burke JF, Bondoc CC. Primary excision and immediate wound closure. Intensive Care Med 1981;7:71–6.

24. Eisenbud D, Huang NF, Luke S, et al. Skin substitutes and wound healing: current status and challenges. Wounds 2004;16:2–17.

25. Hansen SL, Voigt DW, Wiebelhaus P, et al. Using skin replacement products to treat burns and wounds. Adv Skin Wound Care 2001;14:37–44 [quiz: 45-36].

26. Waymack P, Duff RG, Sabolinski M. The effect of a tissue engineered bilayered living skin analog, over meshed split-thickness autografts on the healing of excised burn wounds. The Apligraf Burn Study Group. Burns 2000;26:609–19.

27. Hansbrough JF, Mozingo DW, Kealey GP, et al. Clinical trials of a biosynthetic temporary skin replacement, Dermagraft-Transitional Covering, compared with cryopreserved human cadaver skin for temporary coverage of excised burn wounds. J Burn Care Rehabil 1997;18:43–51.

28. Pham C, Greenwood J, Cleland H, et al. Bio-engineered skin substitutes for the management of burns: a systematic review. Burns 2007;33:946–57.

29. Khachemoune A, Bello YM, Phillips TJ. Factors that influence healing in chronic venous ulcers treated with cryopreserved human epidermal cultures. Dermatol Surg 2002;28:274–80.

30. Alvarez-Diaz C, Cuenca-Pardo J, Sossa-Serrano A. Burns treated with frozen cultured human allogeneic epidermal sheets. J Burn Care Rehabil 2000; 21:291–9.

31. Bolivar-Flores YJ, Kuri-Harcuch W. Frozen allogeneic human epidermal cultured sheets for the cure of complicated leg ulcers. Dermatol Surg 1999;25:610–7.

32. Rheinwald JG, Green H. Serial cultivation of strains of human epidermal keratinocytes: the formation of keratinizing colonies from single cells. Cell 1975;6: 331–43.

33. Bolivar-Flores J, Poumian E, Marsch-Moreno M, et al. Use of cultured human epidermal keratinocytes for allografting burns and conditions for temporary banking of the cultured allografts. Burns 1990;16:3–8.

34. Duinslaeger LA, Verbeken G, Vanhalle S, et al. Cultured allogeneic keratinocyte sheets accelerate healing compared to Op-site treatment of donor sites in burns. J Burn Care Rehabil 1997;18:545–51.

35. Madden MR, LaBruna AA, Hajjar DP, et al. Transplantation of cryopreserved cultured epidermal allografts. J Trauma 1996;40:743–50.

36. Woodley DT, Peterson HD, Herzog SR, et al. Burn wounds resurfaced by cultured epidermal autografts show abnormal reconstitution of anchoring fibrils. JAMA 1988;259:2566–71.

37. Wainwright DJ. Use of an acellular allograft dermal matrix (AlloDerm) in the management of full-thickness burns. Burns 1995;21:243–8.

38. Supp DM, Boyce ST. Engineered skin substitutes: practices and potentials. Clin Dermatol 2005;23: 403–12.

39. Kolokol'chikova EG, Budkevich LI, Bobrovnikov AE, et al. Morphological changes in burn wounds after transplantation of allogenic fibroblasts. Bull Exp Biol Med 2001;131:89–93.

40. Strande LF, Foley ST, Doolin EJ, et al. In vitro bio-artificial skin culture model of tissue rejection and

inflammatory/immune mechanisms. Transplant Proc 1997;29:2118–9.

41. Clark RA, Ghosh K, Tonnesen MG. Tissue engineering for cutaneous wounds. J Invest Dermatol 2007;127:1018–29.

42. Campoccia D, Doherty P, Radice M, et al. Semisynthetic resorbable materials from hyaluronan esterification. Biomaterials 1998;19:2101–27.

43. Caravaggi C, De Giglio R, Pritelli C, et al. HYAFF 11-based autologous dermal and epidermal grafts in the treatment of noninfected diabetic plantar and dorsal foot ulcers: a prospective, multicenter, controlled, randomized clinical trial. Diab Care 2003;26:2853–9.

44. Uccioli L. A clinical investigation on the characteristics and outcomes of treating chronic lower extremity wounds using the TissueTech Autograft System. Int J Low Extrem Wounds 2003;2: 140–51.

45. Myers SR, Grady J, Soranzo C, et al. A hyaluronic acid membrane delivery system for cultured keratinocytes: clinical "take" rates in the porcine keratodermal model. J Burn Care Rehabil 1997;18: 214–22.

46. Nomi M, Atala A, Coppi PD, et al. Principals of neovascularization for tissue engineering. Mol Aspects Med 2002;23:463–83.

47. Eppler SM, Combs DL, Henry TD, et al. A target-mediated model to describe the pharmacokinetics and hemodynamic effects of recombinant human vascular endothelial growth factor in humans. Clin Pharmacol Ther 2002;72:20–32.

48. George ML, Eccles SA, Tutton MG, et al. Correlation of plasma and serum vascular endothelial growth factor levels with platelet count in colorectal cancer: clinical evidence of platelet scavenging? Clin Cancer Res 2000;6:3147–52.

49. Richardson TP, Peters MC, Ennett AB, et al. Polymeric system for dual growth factor delivery. Nat Biotechnol 2001;19:1029–34.

50. Tremblay PL, Hudon V, Berthod F, et al. Inosculation of tissue-engineered capillaries with the host's vasculature in a reconstructed skin transplanted on mice. American journal of transplantation: official journal of the American Society of Transplantation and the American Society of Transplant Surgeons 2005;5:1002–10.

51. Swope VB, Supp AP, Cornelius JR, et al. Regulation of pigmentation in cultured skin substitutes by cytometric sorting of melanocytes and keratinocytes. J Invest Dermatol 1997;109:289–95.

52. Abdel-Malek ZA. Endocrine factors as effectors of integumental pigmentation. Dermatol Clin 1988;6: 175–83.

53. Nordlund JJ, Abdel-Malek ZA, Boissy RE, et al. Pigment cell biology: an historical review. J Invest Dermatol 1989;92:53S–60S.

54. Rogers G, Martinet N, Steinert P, et al. Cultivation of murine hair follicles as organoids in a collagen matrix. J Invest Dermatol 1987;89:369–79.

55. Weinberg WC, Brown PD, Stetler-Stevenson WG, et al. Growth factors specifically alter hair follicle cell proliferation and collagenolytic activity alone or in combination. Differentiation 1990;45:168–78.

56. Philpott MP, Green MR, Kealey T. Human hair growth in vitro. J Cell Sci 1990;97(Pt 3):463–71.

57. Huang Z, Yang J, Luo G, et al. Embryonic porcine skin precursors can successfully develop into integrated skin without teratoma formation posttransplantation in nude mouse model. PLoS ONE 2010;5:e8717.

58. Ohyama M. Hair follicle bulge: a fascinating reservoir of epithelial stem cells. J Dermatol Sci 2007;46: 81–9.

59. Taylor G, Lehrer MS, Jensen PJ, et al. Involvement of follicular stem cells in forming not only the follicle but also the epidermis. Cell 2000;102:451–61.

60. Roh C, Lyle S. Cutaneous stem cells and wound healing. Pediatr Res 2006;59:100R–3R.

61. Huang S, Xu Y, Wu C, et al. In vitro constitution and in vivo implantation of engineered skin constructs with sweat glands. Biomaterials 2010;31:5520–5.

62. Green H. The birth of therapy with cultured cells. BioEssays 2008;30:897–903.

63. Sun T, Jackson S, Haycock JW, et al. Culture of skin cells in 3D rather than 2D improves their ability to survive exposure to cytotoxic agents. J Biotechnol 2006;122:372–81.

64. Robinson MK, Osborne R, Perkins MA. Strategies for the assessment of acute skin irritation potential. J Pharmacol Toxicol Meth 1999;42:1–9.

65. Asselineau D, Bernard B, Bailly C, et al. Human epidermis reconstructed by culture: is it "normal"? J Investig Dermatol 1986;86:181–6.

66. Johnson E, Meunier S, Roy C, et al. Serial cultivation of normal human keratinocytes: a defined system for studying the regulation of growth and differentiation. In Vitro Cell Dev Biol 1992;28:429–35.

67. Boehnke K, Mirancea N, Pavesio A, et al. Effects of fibroblasts and microenvironment on epidermal regeneration and tissue function in long-term skin equivalents. Eur J Cell Biol 2007;86:731–46.

68. El-Ghalbzouri A, Gibbs S, Lamme E, et al. Effect of fibroblasts on epidermal regeneration. Br J Dermatol 2002;147:230–43.

69. Xie Y, Rizzi SC, Dawson R, et al. Development of a three-dimensional human skin equivalent wound model for investigating novel wound healing therapies. Tissue Eng C Meth 2010;16:1111–23.

70. Roguet R. Use of skin cell cultures for in vitro assessment of corrosion and cutaneous irritancy. Cell Biol Toxicol 1999;15:63–75.

71. Welss T, Basketter DA, Schroder KR. In vitro skin irritation: facts and future. State of the art review

of mechanisms and models. Toxicol In Vitro 2004; 18:231–43.

72. Draize J, Woodard G, Calvery H. Methods for the study of irritation and toxicity of substances applied topically to the skin and mucous membranes. J Pharmacol Exp Ther 1944;82:377–90.

73. Campbell RL, Bruce RD. Direct comparison of rabbit and human primary skin irritation responses to isopropylmyristate. Toxicol Appl Pharmacol 1981;563:555–63.

74. Phillips L, et al. A comparison of rabbit and human skin response to certain irritants. Toxicol Appl Pharmacol 1972;21:369–82.

75. EU, Seventh Amendment to the EU Cosmetics Directive 76/768/EEC. In: The European Parliament and the Council of the European Union (Ed.), Brussels, 2003.

76. Becker RA, Borgert CJ, Webb S, et al. Report of an ISRTP workshop: progress and barriers to incorporating alternative toxicological methods in the U.S. Regul Toxicol Pharmacol 2006;46:18–22.

77. EU, Regulation (EC) No 1907/2006, in: E.P.A.T.C.O.T.E. UNION (Ed.), Official Journal of the European Union; 2006. p. L 396/391.

78. Kuroyanagi Y, Kubo K, Matsui H, et al. Establishment of banking system for allogeneic cultured dermal substitute. Artif Organs 2004;28:13–21.

79. Oliver GJ, Pemberton Ma, Rhodes C. An in vitro model for identifying skin-corrosive chemicals. I. Initial validation. Toxicol In Vitro 1988;2:7–17.

80. Scala R, Fentem J, Chen J, et al. Corrositex(r): an in vitro test method for assessing dermal corrosivity potential of chemicals 1999.

81. Stobbe JL, Drake KD, Maier KJ. Comparison of in vivo (Draize method) and in vitro (Corrositex assay) dermal corrosion values for selected industrial chemicals. Int J Toxicol 2003;22:99.

82. Perkins Ma, Osborne R, Johnson GR. Development of an in vitro method for skin corrosion testing. Fundam Appl Toxicol 1996;31:9–18.

83. Fentem J, Archer G, Balls M, et al. The ECVAM international validation study on in vitro tests for skin corrosivity. 2. Results and evaluation by the Management Team. Toxicol in Vitro 1998;12: 483–524.

84. Kandárová H, Liebsch M, Spielmann H, et al. Assessment of the human epidermis model Skin-Ethic RHE for in vitro skin corrosion testing of chemicals according to new OECD TG 431. Toxicol In Vitro 2006;20:547–59.

85. Kidd DA, Johnson M, Clements J. Development of an in vitro corrosion/irritation prediction assay using the EpiDerm skin model. Toxicol In Vitro 2007;21: 1292–7.

86. ECVAM, Statement on the application of the Epi-Derm™ human skin model for skin corrosivity testing, in, 2000.

87. ECVAM, Statement on the application of the Skin-Ethic™ human skin model for skin corrosivity testing, in, 2006.

88. ECVAM, ESAC statement on the scientific validity of an in-vitro test method for skin corrosivity testing, in, 2009.

89. Perkins MA, Osborne R, Rana FR, et al. Comparison of in vitro and in vivo human skin responses to consumer products and ingredients with a range of irritancy potential. Toxicol Sci 1999;48:218–29.

90. Coquette A. Analysis of interleukin-1α (IL-1α) and interleukin-8 (IL-8) expression and release in in vitro reconstructed human epidermis for the prediction of in vivo skin irritation and/or sensitization. Toxicol In Vitro 2003;17:311–21.

91. Shanmugasundaram N, Ravikumar T, Babu M. Comparative physico-chemical and in vitro properties of fibrillated collagen scaffolds from different sources. J Biomater Appl 2004;18:247–64.

92. Ohtani T, Okamoto K, Kaminaka C, et al. Digital gangrene associated with idiopathic hypereosinophilia: treatment with allogeneic cultured dermal substitute (CDS). Eur J Dermatol 2004;14:168–71.

93. Eskes C, Cole T, Hoffmann S, et al. The ECVAM international validation study on in vitro tests for acute skin irritation: selection of test chemicals. Altern Lab Anim 2007;35:603–19.

94. Spielmann H, Hoffmann S, Liebsch M, et al. The ECVAM international validation study on in vitro tests for acute skin irritation: report on the validity of the EPISKIN and EpiDerm assays and on the Skin Integrity Function Test. Altern Lab Anim 2007;35:559–601.

95. Gabbanini S, Lucchi E, Carli M, et al. In vitro evaluation of the permeation through reconstructed human epidermis of essentials oils from cosmetic formulations. J Pharm Biomed Anal 2009;50: 370–6.

96. Jager MD, Groenink W, Spek JVD, et al. Preparation and characterization of a stratum corneum substitute for in vitro percutaneous penetration studies, 1758 (2006) 636–644.

97. Gysler A, Kleuser B, Sippl W, et al. Skin penetration and metabolism of topical glucocorticoids in reconstructed epidermis and in excised human skin. Pharm Res 1999;16:1386–91.

98. Ackermann K, Lombardi Borgia S, Korting H, et al. The Phenion(r) full-thickness skin model for percutaneous absorption testing. Skin Pharmacol Physiol 2009;23:105–12.

99. Bouwstra JA, Ponec M. The skin barrier in healthy and diseased state. Wide Angle Q. J. Film Hist. Theory Criticism Pract 2006;1758:2080–95.

100. Scheuplein RJ. Mechanism of percutaneous absorption. II. Transient diffusion and the relative importance of various routes of skin penetration. J Invest Dermatol 1967;48:79–88.

101. Kao J, Hall J, Helman G. *In vitro* percutaneous absorption in mouse skin: influence of skin appendages. Toxicol Appl Pharmacol 1988;94:93–103.

102. Illel B, Schaefer H, Wepierre J, et al. Follicles play an important role in percutaneous absorption. J Pharm Sci 1991;80:424–7.

103. Michel M, L'Heureux N, Pouliot R, et al. Characterization of a new tissue-engineered human skin equivalent with hair. In Vitro Cell Dev Biol Anim 1999;35:318–26.

104. Brenner M, Hearing VJ. The protective role of melanin against UV damage in human skin. Photochem Photobiol 2008;84:539–49.

105. Chen G, Sato T, Ohgushi H, et al. Culturing of skin fibroblasts in a thin PLGA-collagen hybrid mesh. Biomaterials 2005;26:2559–66.

106. Bertaux B, Morliere P, Moreno G, et al. Growth of melanocytes in a skin equivalent model *in vitro*. Br J Dermatol 1988;119:503–12.

107. Bessou S, Surléve-Bazeille JE, Sorbier E, et al. *Ex vivo* reconstruction of the epidermis with melanocytes and the influence of UVB. Pigment Cell 1995;8:241–9.

108. Topol BM, Haimes HB, Dubertret L, et al. Transfer of melanosomes in a skin equivalent model *in vitro*. J Invest Dermatol 1986;87:642–7.

109. Bernerd F, Asselineau D. Successive alteration and recovery of epidermal differentiation and morphogenesis after specific UVB-damages in skin reconstructed *in vitro*. Dev Biol 1997;183:123–38.

110. Maresca V, Flori E, Briganti S, et al. UVA-induced modification of catalase charge properties in the epidermis is correlated with the skin phototype. J Investig Dermatol 2006;126:182–90.

111. Garibyan L, Fisher DE. How sunlight causes melanoma. Curr Oncol Rep 2010;12:319–26.

112. Bernerd F, Asselineau D. An organotypic model of skin to study photodamage and photoprotection *in vitro*. J Am Acad Dermatol 2008;58:S155–9.

113. Leliàvre D, Justine P, Christiaens F, et al. The episkin phototoxicity assay (EPA): development of an *in vitro* tiered strategy using 17 reference chemicals to predict phototoxic potency. Toxicol. In Vitro 2007;21:977–95.

114. Nolte SV, Xu W, Rennekampff H-O, et al. Diversity of fibroblasts–a review on implications for skin tissue engineering. Cells Tissues Organs 2008;187:165–76.

115. Freshney RI. Culture of Animal Cells. In: A Manual of Basic Techniques. New York: Wiley & Liss; 2000.

116. Falanga V, Isaacs C, Paquette D, et al. Wounding of bioengineered skin: cellular and molecular aspects after injury. J Investig Dermatol 2002;119:653–60.

117. Andriani F, Margulis A, Lin N, et al. Analysis of microenvironmental factors contributing to basement membrane assembly and normalized epidermal phenotype. J Investig Dermatol 2003;120:923–31.

118. Lee D-Y, Cho K-H. The effects of epidermal keratinocytes and dermal fibroblasts on the formation of cutaneous basement membrane in three-dimensional culture systems. Arch Dermatol Res 2005;296:296–302.

119. Maas-Szabowski N, Shimotoyodome A, Fusenig NE. Keratinocyte growth regulation in fibroblast cocultures via a double paracrine mechanism. J Cell Sci 1999;112(Pt 1):1843–53.

120. Maas-Szabowski N, Stark HJ, Fusenig NE. Keratinocyte growth regulation in defined organotypic cultures through IL-1-induced keratinocyte growth factor expression in resting fibroblasts. J Investig Dermatol 2000;114:1075–84.

121. Coulomb B, Dubertet L, Merrill C, et al. The collagen lattice: a model for studying the physiology, biosynthetic function and pharmacology of the skin. Br J Dermatol 1984;111(Suppl 27):83–7.

122. Bell E, Ehrlich HP, Buttle DJ, et al. Living tissue formed *in vitro* and accepted as skin-equivalent tissue of full thickness. Science (New York, NY) 1981;211:1052–4.

123. Sun T, Jackson S, Haycock JW, et al. Culture of skin cells in 3D rather than 2D improves their ability to survive exposure to cytotoxic agents. J Biotechnol 2006;122:372–81.

124. Bell E, Sher S, Hull B, et al. The reconstitution of living skin. J Investig 1983;81(1 Suppl):2s–10s.

125. Laska DA, Poulsen RG, Horn JW, et al. An evaluation of TESTSKIN™: an alternative dermal irritation model. In Vitro Toxicol 1992;5:177–89.

126. Parenteau NL, Bilbo P, Nolte CJ, et al. The organotypic culture of human skin keratinocytes and fibroblasts to achieve form and function. Cytotechnology 1992;9:163–71.

127. Stark H-J, Boehnke K, Mirancea N, et al. Epidermal homeostasis in long-term scaffold-enforced skin equivalents. J Investig Dermatol Symp Proc 2006;11:93–105.

128. Sahuc F, Nakazawa K, Berthod F. Mesenchymal-epithelial interactions regulate gene expression of type V11 collagen and kalinin in keratinocytes and dermal-epidermal junction formation in a skin equivalent model. Wound Repair Regen 1996;4:93–102.

129. Lindberg K, Badylak SF. Porcine small intestinal submucosa (SIS): a bioscaffold supporting *in vitro* primary human epidermal cell differentiation and synthesis of basement membrane proteins. Burns 2001;27:254–66.

130. Ng KW, Hutmacher DW. Reduced contraction of skin equivalent engineered using cell sheets cultured in 3D matrices. Biomaterials 2006;27:4591–8.

131. Bruin P, Smedinga J, Pennings AJ, et al. Biodegradable lysine diisocyanate-based poly(glycolide-co-epsilon-caprolactone)-urethane network in artificial skin. Biomaterials 1990;11:291–5.

132. Ng KW, Khor HL, Hutmacher DW. *In vitro* characterization of natural and synthetic dermal matrices cultured with human dermal fibroblasts. Biomaterials 2004;25:2807–18.

133. Dai NT, Yeh MK, Chiang CH, et al. Human single-donor composite skin substitutes based on collagen and polycaprolactone copolymer. Biochem Biophys Res Commun 2009;386:21–5.

134. Graf R, Kock M, Bock A, et al. Lipophilic prodrugs of amino acids and vitamin E as osmolytes for the compensation of hyperosmotic stress in human keratinocytes. Exp Dermatol 2009;18:370–7.

135. Williams IR, Kupper TS. Immunity at the surface: homeostatic mechanisms of the skin immune system. Life Sci 1996;58:1485–507.

136. Régnier M, Staquet MJ, Schmitt D, et al. Integration of Langerhans cells into a pigmented reconstructed human epidermis. In: The Journal of investigative dermatology; p. 510–2.

137. Fransson J, Heffler LC, Tengvall Linder M, et al. Culture of human epidermal Langerhans cells in a skin equivalent. Br J Dermatol 1998;139:598–604.

138. Boyce ST. Cultured skin substitutes: a review. Tissue Eng 1996;2:255–66.

139. Koblizek TI, Weiss C, Yancopoulos GD, et al. Angiopoietin-1 induces sprouting angiogenesis *in vitro*. Curr Biol 1998;8:529–32.

140. Nör JE, Christensen J, Mooney DJ, et al. Vascular endothelial growth factor (VEGF)-mediated angiogenesis is associated with enhanced endothelial cell survival and induction of Bcl-2 expression. Am J Pathol 1999;154:375–84.

141. Trochon V, Li H, Vasse M, et al. Endothelial metalloprotease-disintegrin protein (ADAM) is implicated in angiogenesis *in vitro*. Angiogenesis 1998;2:277–85.

142. Bach TL, Barsigian C, Yaen CH, et al. Endothelial cell VE-cadherin functions as a receptor for the beta15-42 sequence of fibrin. J Biol Chem 1998;273:30719–28.

143. Bayless KJ, Salazar R, Davis GE. RGD-dependent vacuolation and lumen formation observed during endothelial cell morphogenesis in three-dimensional fibrin matrices involves the alpha(v)beta(3) and alpha(5)beta(1) integrins. Am J Pathol 2000;156:1673–83.

144. Black AF, Berthod F, L'Heureux N, et al. *In vitro* reconstruction of a human capillary-like network in a tissue-engineered skin equivalent. FASEB J 1998;12:1331–40.

145. Donovan D, Brown NJ, Bishop ET, et al. Comparison of three *in vitro* human 'angiogenesis' assays with capillaries formed *in vivo*. Angiogenesis 2001;4:113–21.

146. Ponec M, El Ghalbzouri A, Dijkman R, et al. Endothelial network formed with human dermal microvascular endothelial cells in autologous multicellular skin substitutes. Angiogenesis 2004;7:295–305.

147. Dewey CF Jr, Bussolari SR, Gimbrone MA Jr, et al. The dynamic response of vascular endothelial cells to fluid shear stress. J Biomech Eng 1981;103:177–85.

148. Bandarchi B, Ma L, Navab R, et al. From melanocyte to metastatic malignant melanoma. Dermatol. Res. Pract 2010. Article ID 583748, 8 pages, doi:10.1155/2010/583748.

149. Bowcock AM, Krueger JG. Getting under the skin: the immunogenetics of psoriasis. Nat Rev Immunol 2005;5:699–711.

150. Danilenko DM. Review paper: preclinical models of psoriasis. Vet Pathol 2008;45:563–75.

151. Saiag P, Coulomb B, Lebreton C, et al. Psoriatic fibroblasts induce hyperproliferation of normal keratinocytes in a skin equivalent model *in vitro*. Science 1985;230:669–72.

152. Fransson J, Hammar H, Emilson A, et al. Proliferation and interferon-γ receptor expression in psoriatic and healthy keratinocytes are influenced by interactions between keratinocytes and fibroblasts in a skin equivalent model. Arch Dermatol Res 1995;287:517–23.

153. Konstantinova NV, Duong DM, Remenyik E, et al. Interleukin-8 is induced in skin equivalents and is highest in those derived from psoriatic fibroblasts. J Invest Dermatol 1996;107:615–21.

154. Baker BS, Griffiths CE, Lambert S, et al. The effects of cyclosporin A on T lymphocyte and dendritic cell sub-populations in psoriasis. Br J Dermatol 1987;116:503–10.

155. Prinz J, Braun-Falco O, Meurer M, et al. Chimaeric CD4 monoclonal antibody in treatment of generalised pustular psoriasis. Lancet 1991;320–1.

156. Gottlieb S, Gilleaudeau P, Johnson R, et al. Response of psoriasis to a lymphocyte-selective toxin (DAB389IL-2) suggests a primary immune, but not keratinocyte, pathogenic basis. Nat Med 1995;1:442–7.

157. Jean J, Lapointe M, Soucy J, et al. Development of an *in vitro* psoriatic skin model by tissue engineering. J Dermatol Sci 2009;53:19–25.

158. Barker CL, McHale MT, Gillies AK, et al. The development and characterization of an *in vitro* model of psoriasis. J Investig Dermatol 2004;123:892–901.

159. Harrison CA, Layton CM, Hau Z, et al. Transglutaminase inhibitors induce hyperproliferation and parakeratosis in tissue-engineered skin. Br J Dermatol 2007;156:247–57.

160. Tjabringa G, Bergers M, van Rens D, et al. Development and validation of human psoriatic skin equivalents. Am J Pathol 2008;173:815–23.

161. Kalish RS, Simon M, Harrington R, et al. Skin equivalent and natural killer cells: a new model for psoriasis and GVHD. J Invest Dermatol 2009;129:773–6.

162. Uong A, Zon LI. Melanocytes in development and cancer. J Cell Physiol 2010;222:38–41.

163. Hsu M-Y, Meier F, Herlyn M. Melanoma development and progression: a conspiracy between tumor and host. Differentiation 2002;70:522–36.

164. Shih IM, Elder DE, Hsu MY, et al. Regulation of Mel-CAM/MUC18 expression on melanocytes of different stages of tumor progression by normal keratinocytes. Am J Pathol 1994;145:837–45.

165. Walles T, Weimer M, Linke K, et al. The potential of bioartificial tissues in oncology research and treatment. Onkologie 2007;30:388–94.

166. Meier F, Nesbit M, Hsu MY, et al. Human melanoma progression in skin reconstructs: biological significance of bFGF. Am J Pathol 2000;156:193–200.

167. Eves P, Haycock J, Layton C, et al. Anti-inflammatory and anti-invasive effects of alpha-melanocyte-stimulating hormone in human melanoma cells. Br J Cancer 2003;89:2004–15.

168. Eves P, Katerinaki E, Simpson C, et al. Melanoma invasion in reconstructed human skin is influenced by skin cells–investigation of the role of proteolytic enzymes. Clin Exp Metastasis 2003;20:685–700.

169. Van Kilsdonk JWJ, Bergers M, Van Kempen LCLT, et al. Keratinocytes drive melanoma invasion in a reconstructed skin model. Melanoma Res 2010; 20:372.

170. Gaggioli C, Robert G, Bertolotto C, et al. Tumor-derived fibronectin is involved in melanoma cell invasion and regulated by V600E B-Raf signaling pathway. J Investig Dermatol 2007;127:400–10.

171. Grindon C, Combes R, Cronin MT, et al. A review of the status of alternative approaches to animal testing and the development of integrated testing strategies for assessing the toxicity of chemicals under REACH–a summary of a DEFRA-funded project conducted by Liverpool John Moores University. Altern Lab Anim 2006;34:149–458.

172. Meier F, Busch S, Lasithiotakis K, et al. Combined targeting of MAPK and AKT signalling pathways is a promising strategy for melanoma treatment. Br J Dermatol 2007;156:1204–13.

173. Folkman J. What is the evidence that tumors are angiogenesis dependent? J Natl Cancer Inst 1990;82:4–6.

174. Liotta LA, Kleinerman J, Saidel GM. Quantitative relationships of intravascular tumor cells, tumor vessels, and pulmonary metastases following tumor implantation. Cancer Res 1974;34:997–1004.

175. Weiss SJ. Tissue destruction by neutrophils. N Engl J Med 1989;320:365–76.

176. Martin P, Leibovich SJ. Inflammatory cells during wound repair: the good, the bad and the ugly. Trends Cell Biol 2005;15:599–607.

177. Leibovich SJ, Ross R. The role of the macrophage in wound repair. A study with hydrocortisone and anti-macrophage serum. Am J Pathol 1975;78:71–100.

178. Polverini PJ, Cotran PS, Gimbrone MA Jr, et al. Activated macrophages induce vascular proliferation. Nature 1977;269:804–6.

179. Eming SA, Brachvogel B, Odorisio T, et al. Regulation of angiogenesis: wound healing as a model. Prog Histochem Cytochem 2007;42:115–70.

180. Coolen NA, Vlig M, van den Bogaerdt AJ, et al. Development of an in vitro burn wound model. Wound Repair Regen 2008;16:559–67.

181. Schreier T, Degen E, Baschong W. Fibroblast migration and proliferation during in vitro wound healing. A quantitative comparison between various growth factors and a low molecular weight blood dialysate used in the clinic to normalize impaired wound healing. Res Exp Med (Berl) 1993;193:195–205.

182. Kratz G. Modeling of wound healing processes in human skin using tissue culture. Microsc Res Tech 1998;42:345–50.

183. Emanuelsson P, Kratz G. Characterization of a new in vitro burn wound model. Burns 1997;23:32–6.

184. Vaughan MB, Ramirez RD, Brown SA, et al. A reproducible laser-wounded skin equivalent model to study the effects of aging in vitro. Rejuvenation Res 2004;7:99–110.

185. Mishra NN, Prasad T, Sharma N, et al. Pathogenicity and drug resistance in Candida albicans and other yeast species. A review. Acta Microbiol Immunol Hung 2007;54:201–35.

186. Green CB. RT-PCR detection of Candida albicans ALS gene expression in the reconstituted human epithelium (RHE) model of oral candidiasis and in model biofilms. Microbiology 2004;150:267–75.

187. Schaller M, Preidel H, Januschke E, et al. Light and electron microscopic findings in a model of human cutaneous candidosis based on reconstructed human epidermis following the topical application of different econazole formulations. J Drug Target 1999;6:361–72.

188. Korting HC, Patzak U, Schaller M, et al. A model of human cutaneous candidosis based on reconstructed human epidermis for the light and electron microscopic study of pathogenesis and treatment. J Infect 1998;36:259–67.

189. Schaller M, Mailhammer R, Korting HC. Cytokine expression induced by Candida albicans in a model of cutaneous candidosis based on reconstituted human epidermis. J Med Microbiol 2002; 51:672–6.

190. Schaller M, Schackert C, Korting HC, et al. Invasion of Candida albicans correlates with expression of secreted aspartic proteinases during experimental infection of human epidermis. J Investig Dermatol 2000;114:712–7.

191. Korting HC, Schaller M, Eder G, et al. Effects of the human immunodeficiency virus (HIV) proteinase inhibitors saquinavir and indinavir on in vitro activities

of secreted aspartyl proteinases of *Candida albicans* isolates from HIV-infected patients. Antimicrob Agents Chemother 1999;43:2038–42.

192. Andrei G, Duraffour S, Van den Oord J, et al. Epithelial raft cultures for investigations of virus growth, pathogenesis and efficacy of antiviral agents. Antivir Res 2010;85:431–49.

193. Riediger C, Sauer P, Matevossian E, et al. Herpes simplex virus sepsis and acute liver failure. Clin Transplant 2009;23:37–41.

194. Tabbara KF, Al Balushi N. Topical ganciclovir in the treatment of acute herpetic keratitis. Clin. Ophthalmol (Auckland, NZ) 2010;4:905–12.

195. Stevens JG, Cook ML. Latent herpes simplex virus in spinal ganglia of mice. Science 1971;173:843–5.

196. Visalli RJ, Courtney RJ, Meyers C. Infection and replication of herpes simplex virus type 1 in an organotypic epithelial culture system. Virology 1997; 230:236–43.

197. Hukkanen V, Mikola H, Nykänen M, et al. Herpes simplex virus type 1 infection has two separate modes of spread in three-dimensional keratinocyte culture. J Gen Virol 1999;80(Pt 8):2149–55.

198. Syrjänen S, Mikola H, Nykänen M, et al. *In vitro* establishment of lytic and nonproductive infection by herpes simplex virus type 1 in three-dimensional keratinocyte culture. J Virol 1996;70:6524–8.

199. Andrei G, Oord JVD, Fiten P, et al. Organotypic epithelial raft cultures as a model for evaluating compounds against alphaherpesviruses. Society 2005;49:4671–80.

200. Penfold ME, Armati P, Cunningham AL. Axonal transport of herpes simplex virions to epidermal cells: evidence for a specialized mode of virus transport and assembly. Proc Natl Acad Sci USA 1994;91:6529–33.

201. Tfayli A, Piot O, Draux F, et al. Molecular characterization of reconstructed skin model by Raman microspectroscopy: comparison with excised human skin. Biopolymers 2007;87:261–74.

202. Allen-Hoffmann BL, Schlosser SJ, Ivarie CAR, et al. Normal growth and differentiation in a spontaneously immortalized near-diploid human keratinocyte cell line, NIKS. Differentiation 2000;444–55.

203. Marston WA, Hanft J, Norwood P, et al. The efficacy and safety of Dermagraft in improving the healing of chronic diabetic foot ulcers: results of a prospective randomized trial. Diab Care 2003; 26:1701–5.

204. Dieterich C, Schandar M, Noll M, et al. In vitro reconstructed human epithelia reveal contributions of Candida albicans EFG1 and CPH1 to adhesion and invasion. Microbiology 2002 Feb;148(Pt 2): 497–506.

Pre- and Probiotics for Human Skin

Jean Krutmann

KEYWORD

- Pre- and probiotics for human skin

INTRODUCTION

Prebiotics have been defined as "non-digestible food ingredients that beneficially affect the host by selectively stimulating the growth and/or activity of one, or a limiting number of, bacteria in the colon".[1] This concept has originally been developed for the gut, but in principle can be applied to modulate the composition of any microbial community including the skin microflora to achieve beneficial effects.

Scientific interest in the composition and function of the skin's microflora (=the skin's microbiota) is currently experiencing a revival, and in fact, has become one of the most exciting and rapidly developing areas in cutaneous biology.[2] A major driving force for this development has been the discovery that epidermal keratinocytes have the potential to affect the cutaneous microflora by producing antimicrobial peptides.[3] Also, recent research efforts to understand the control of skin barrier functions unambiguously point to a close link between physical, immunological and cell biological properties of the skin and its microflora.[4,5] Manipulation of the composition and/or function of the skin microflora by prebiotic strategies, which, in contrast to antibiotics, may allow selective inhibition of detrimental and at the same time preservation and/or stimulation of beneficial bacteria, is therefore of obvious interest in dermatology.[2]

In contrast to prebiotics, probiotics are based on the use of living organisms which upon ingestion in certain numbers exert health beneficial effects beyond inherent general nutrition.[6] Probiotics have been widely used for the treatment/prevention of gastrointestinal disorders, but a growing number of clinical studies suggest that probiotic strategies induce systemic effects which extend beyond the gut and may even affect selected functions of the skin.[7] Accordingly, modulation of the gut's microflora through probiotics appears to cause beneficial effects in healthy as well as diseased human skin.[8,9]

This article briefly summarizes the scientific basis for such strategies and provides a critical overview about the currently available studies on the use of pre- and/or probiotica in clinical dermatology and cosmetics.

MICROFLORA OF HUMAN SKIN

The normal human skin microflora is composed of a limited number of microbial types, as outlined below. This is a direct consequence of the unique environmental conditions the skin offers to microbes, which markedly differ from those found at mucosal surfaces. In other words only a limited number of microbial types (mainly Gram-positive species) have evolved to take advantage of the harsh environmental conditions that are being offered by the skin.[10]

In general, resident and transient microbial species are present on the skin. The term resident refers to viable, reproducing populations, whereas transient species are defined as contaminants with little or no capacity for sustained growth and reproduction in the cutaneous environment. Resident microbial species include *Proprionibacteria* (*P acnes*, *P avidum* and *P granulosum*), Coagulase-negative *Staphylococci* (*Staphylococcus epidermidis*), *Micrococci*, *Corynebacteria*

This article originally published in *Journal of Dermatological Science 54 (2009) 1–5*, Elsevier.
Institut für Umweltmedizinische Forschung (IUF) at the Heinrich-Heine-University, Düsseldorf gGmbH, Auf'm Hennekamp 50, D-4025 Düsseldorf, Germany
E-mail address: krutmann@rz.uni-duesseldorf.de

plasticsurgery.theclinics.com

and *Acinetobacter*. In addition, there are Malassezia yeast species and a variety of bacteriophage species. Common transient species are *Staphylococcus aureus*, *Escherichia coli*, *Pseudomonas aeroguinosa* and *Bacillus* species. It should be emphasized that the above said represents the "textbook" knowledge on the skin's microflora, which is limited to culture-dependent assays, although it is estimated that less than 1% of harvested species can be cultivated. More recent studies employing 16SrRNA gene survey strategies indicate that the human skin microbiota is far more complex[11,12] and in fact comprises 113 phylotypes that belong to six bacterial divisions. Among these, Proteobacteria dominate the skin microbiota. In contrast, 16 SrRNA sequences that closely match *S epidermidis* and *P acnes* consisted of less than 6% of the captured microbiota. This is in clear contrast to the commonly held notion that *S epidermidis* is the dominant aerobic bacteria resident in skin.[11]

The resident microflora fills a niche that could otherwise be colonized by pathogenic microorganisms that are aggressive and cause infection, either at the skin site or by transfer to other sites. Also, if the skin could be colonized by pathogens adopted for other sites (eg, mucous membranes), this could facilitate the spread of pathogens by offering them more dispersed routes.

This is, however, not the only positive function of the resident microflora. Accordingly, Propionibacteria have been shown to have adjuvant and antitumor activities and to contribute to a more efficient immunological response to general infections.[13,14] On the other hand, the same species are of pathogenic relevance in acne and folliculitis.[15] In aggregate, preservation of the resident microflora is thought to be an effective way to achieve maintenance of healthy "normal" skin functions. It is only when the host becomes compromised by trauma, injury or changes in the immune defense that the resident microflora displays pathogenic potential. Under such circumstances, pathogenic effects not only are restricted to *S epidermidis*, but may also be observed with *Propionibacterium* species. Thus, the resident microflora may be regarded as "beneficial" to the "normal, healthy" host, but may become dangerous to the host with disturbed skin integrity.

The limited number of microbial species that colonize human skin is determined by a variety of physical and biochemical factors.[10,16] The physical factors are mainly defined by the host environment and include the number and size of follicles and glands, gland function, the flow of secretions, the integrity of barrier function, skin pH and osmotic potential. A slightly acidic pH, eg, favors

Proprionibacterium spp., whereas neutral and alkaline pH favors most other resident bacteria. Also, high hydration is associated with higher pH, which is again associated with high microbial population density, eg, in the foot. Biochemical factors include chemical compounds such as soluble micronutrients derived from sebum (lipids and aminoacids) and sweat (vitamins, lactate and amino acids) as well as biochemical molecules which are produced as a consequence of the metabolic activity of microorganisms on the skin and which in turn function to influence colonization. Examples of microbial metabolites controlling other residents are lantibiotics produced by *Staphylococcus* spp. Other factors are methantiol, bacteriocins, organic acids and lytic enzymes, including those produced by bacteriophages. Also, bacterial metabolism affects pH and osmotic potential.

Another level of complexity is provided by the interplay between skin microorganisms and the skin immune system. The skin possesses the capacity to mount both, adaptive and non-adaptive immune responses. Non-adaptive (=innate) immune responses are immediate and non-specific, whereas adaptive immune responses are secondary and selective in nature.

There is currently no evidence to suggest that adaptive immune responses of the skin influence the normal skin microflora. There is, however, some evidence that the skin microflora activates the adaptive immune system. Accordingly, microorganisms on the skin have been shown to be coated with immunoglobulins which are most likely derived from eccrine gland secretions.[17,18] Also, numerous reports have described humoral and cell-mediated immune responses in the peripheral blood against skin microbials (eg,[19–23]). These studies did not clarify, however, whether stimulation of the adaptive immune system occurred via the skin or at a different site where the same or related species of microorganisms reside. In favor of first possibility is the observation that in pityriaisis versicolor, seborrheic dermatitis and dandruff, the immune response to Malassezia species is maintained at higher levels as compared to healthy control subjects.[14,24] Similar observations have also been made in acne patients for immune response against *P acnes*.[25]

In marked contrast to adaptive immune responses, non-adaptive, innate immune responses of the skin are clearly involved in the control of microbial colonization. Accordingly, upon activation by microorganisms, epidermal keratinocytes have the capacity to produce all four known β-defensins as well as cathelicidin hCAP-18 and by producing these antimicrobial peptides inhibit growth or kill microorganisms, i.e. bacteria and also viruses.

A detailed review of the relative importance of these factors and their complex interplay can be found in Reference.[26] In the context of this review it is important to state that skin microflora, skin barrier function and the skin immune system are closely linked to each other and appear to form a complex and highly regulated network that controls a variety of fundamental skin functions. It is therefore no surprise that attempts have been made beyond antibiotica to selectively manipulate this system in order to achieve beneficial effects for human skin.

PREBIOTICS AND SKIN

As outlined above the composition of the skin microflora depends on numerous factors and thus the bacterial equilibrium can easily be disturbed. A prominent example is skin of acne patients where overgrowth of P acnes has been observed.[15] Conventional cosmetic strategies to correct this problem not only make use of antibacterial agents which are effective in reducing the amount of P acnes, but at the same time also affect other, beneficial bacteria such as S epidermidis, which is regarded as a commensal bacterium that serves to protect human skin from infections and other environmental insults, as outlined before. In this regard, a prebiotic strategy that would rebalance the composition of the skin's microflora by inhibiting the growth of P acnes and at the same time preserving the growth of beneficial bacteria seems preferable (**Fig. 1**). Accordingly, recent studies demonstrate the successful development of a prebiotic cosmetic approach to balance the composition of the cutaneous microflora. In these studies skin microflora was analyzed by fluorescence in situ hybridization.[27] This very precise method avoids the drawbacks of cultural methods and allows the direct observation of bacteria on the skin.[28] It was observed that twice daily application of a cosmetic product containing selected plant extracts from either Ginseng or Black currant or pine to human skin for a total of three weeks was effective in inhibiting the growth of P acnes, whereas coagulase negative staphylococci were not affected.[27] This study thus demonstrates that it is generally feasible to improve the composition of the skin microflora, ie, to limit or reduce the growth of pathogenic species and at the same time to preserve or even stimulate the growth of beneficial bacteria. In this regard, such a prebiotic cosmetic approach is clearly superior to antibacterial cosmetic products which unselectively reduce bacterial growth by means of antibiotics or antimicrobial agents.[29] It should be kept in mind, however, that the design of this study was open and the number of volunteers was limited to 11. Further studies are therefore clearly needed to confirm these preliminary observations.

It will also be of interest to access whether and how colonization of human skin with "beneficial" bacteria such as S epidermidis causes beneficial effects in human skin that extend beyond the prevention of overgrowth of human skin by pathogenic bacteria. Theoretically, the presence of S epidermidis could affect the skin barrier function and/or the development of innate immune responses in human skin. Such a bidirectional relationship between the skin and its microflora would provide the basis for the development of prebiotic strategies for the treatment of skin diseases with known deficiencies in barrier function and innate immunity such as atopic eczema.[30]

PROBIOTICS AND SKIN

In contrast to the very limited number of studies on the use of prebiotic strategies in cosmetic and

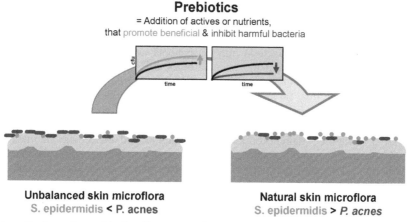

Fig. 1. Topical application of a prebiotic will promote the growth of beneficial and inhibit harmful bacteria.

dermatology, a constantly growing body of the literature exists about the relevance of probiotics for skin. It is now generally believed that probiotics exert beneficial effects by improving the characteristics of the intestinal microflora. Most studies have used lactic acid bacteria, ie, lactobacilli, enterococci and bifidobacteria, that are able to survive through the stomach and small intestine.[7] Probiotic lactic acid bacteria have been linked to many effects including improving rates of recovery from gastroenteritis and diarrhoea of viral and bacterial origins.[31–34] They have been suggested to modulate immunity in the gut but also systemically, and the latter property may be of relevance for human skin.[35] Accordingly, a significant improvement on the course of atopic dermatitis has been reported in infants given probiotic-supplemented elimination diets.[36–39] Also, probiotics administered pre- and postnatally for 6 months may be able to reduce the prevalence of atopic eczema in children at high risk for atopic diseases as compared with placebo treatment,[8] although this preventive effect of probiotics is controversial.[40] The mechanistic basis of skin effects induced by probiotic gut flora is thought to be represented by changes in systemic immune responses. In particular, modulation of specific T-cell subsets such as stimulation of TH1 cells in the gut mucosa which may subsequently influence immune responses in other tissues may play a role.[41–43] Also, in mice, oral administration of *Lactobacillus casei* reduced contact hypersensitivity to a hapten only in the presence of CD4+ T-cells, which control the size of the CD8+ effector pool.[44]

It has been speculated that not only diseased, but also healthy skin may profit from the oral ingestion of probiotic bacteria (**Fig. 2**). Accordingly, nutritional supplementation of hairless mice with *Lactobacillus johnsonii* provided protection of the skin immune system against ultraviolet B radiation-induced immunosuppressive effects.[45] Similar effects have recently been described in a human in vivo study and it has been proposed that oral consumption of probiotic bacteria may represent a novel approach to protect the skin immune system against ultraviolet radiation.[46] Another target for probiotics may be skin barrier function. A recent double-blind, randomized clinical study has shown that a 24-week skin nutrition intervention with a fermented dairy product in female volunteers having dry and sensitive, but otherwise healthy skin significantly reduced transepidermal water loss and thus improved stratum corneum barrier function compared to a placebo product.[47] It should be noted, however, that in addition to the probiotic strains (*L casei, Lactobacillus*

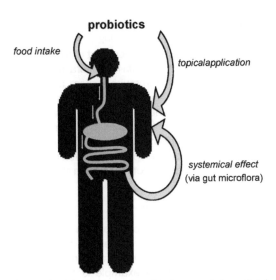

Fig. 2. Oral ingestion of probiotics exerts beneficial effects on the skin through mechanisms which are presumably initiated in the gut. Alternatively, after topical application, probiotics may directly act on skin.

bulgaris and *Stretococcus thermophilus*) this dairy product contained a mixture of boretsch oil, green tea polyphenols and vitamin E and that skin barrier improvement may be at least in part due to these ingredients.

All these approaches have been based on the oral application of probiotic strains. There is, however, at least circumstantial evidence that beneficial effects can also be achieved by topical application of probiotic bacteria to human skin (see **Fig. 2**). In general, nonintestinal applications of probiotics are few and have thus far mainly been used for the urogenital tract There are currently only a very few studies pursuing a probiotic approach for the skin microflora. In this regard,[48] point out the difficulty to identify useful bacteria in view of the harsh environmental conditions that may prevent colonization of skin with a probiotic strain. Nevertheless, results from two studies suggest that topical application of *Vitreoscilla filiformis* exerts beneficial effects in patients with seborrheic dermatitis and atopic eczema.[49,50] *V filiformis* is a Gram-negative bacteria found in thermal spa water from LaRoche-Posay, France, and classically used for dermatological treatment. Although the precise mechanisms through which *V filiformis* improves skin symptoms in atopic and seborrheic dermatitis are not yet known it is tempting to speculate that immunomodulatory effects are at least partially involved. This assumption is supported by very recent studies indicating that *V filiformis* has profound effects on the skin immune system (T. Biedermann, personal communication).

ACKNOWLEDGMENTS

This work has been supported by the Deutsche Forschungsgemeinschaft SFB 728 and GRK 1033.

REFERENCES

1. Gibson GR, Roberfroid MB. Dietary modulation of the human conic micribiota: introducing the concept of prebiotics. J Nutr 1995;125:1401–12.
2. Cogen AL, Nizet V, Gallo RL. Skin microbiota: a source of disease or defense? Brit J Dermatol 2008;158:442–55.
3. Gallo RL, Murakami M, Ohtake T, et al. Biology and clinical relevance of naturally occurring antimicrobial peptides. J Allergy Clin Immunol 2002;110:823–31.
4. Ellias PM. Stratum corneum defensive functions: an integrated view. J Invest Dermatol 2005;125:183–200.
5. Elias PM, Choi EH. Interactions among stratum cormeum defensive functions. Exp Dermatol 2005;14:719–26.
6. Guarner F, Schaafsma GJ. Probiotis. Int J Food Microbiol 1998;39:237–8.
7. Ouwehand AC, Salminen S, Isolauri E. Probiotics: an overview of beneficial effects. Antonie van Leuwenhoek 2002;82:279–89.
8. Kalliomäki M, Salminen S, Arvilommi H, et al. Probiotics in primary prevention of atopic disease: a randomized placebo-controlled trial. Lancet 2001;357:1076–9.
9. Guenche A, Benyacoub J, Buetler TM, et al. Supplementation with oral probiotic bacteria maintains cutaneous immune homeostasis after UV exposure. Eur J Dermatol 2006;16:511–7.
10. Leyden JJ, McGinley KJ, Nordstrom KM, et al. Skin microflora. J Invest Dermatol 1987;88:65s–72s.
11. Grice EA, Kong HH, Renaud G, et al. A diversity profile of the human skin microbiota. Genome Res 2008;18:1043–50.
12. Gao Z, Tseng C, Strober BE, et al. Substantial alterations of the cutaneous bacterial biota in psoriatic lesions. PLoS ONE 2008;3:e2719.
13. Roskowski W, Roskowski K, Ko HL, et al. Immunomodulation by propionibacteria. Zentralblatt für Bakteriologie 1990;274:289–98.
14. Eady EA, Ingham E. Propionibacterium acnes— friend or foe? Rev Med Microbiol 1994;5:163–73.
15. Leyden JJ, McGinley KJ, Bowels B. Propionibacterium acnes colonization in acne and nonacne. Dermatology 1998;196:55–8.
16. Bojar RA, Holland KT. Review: the human cutaneous microflora and factors controlling colonization. World J Microbiol Biotechnol 2002;18:889–903.
17. Okada T, Konishi H, Ito M, et al. Identification of secretory immunoglobulin A in human sweat and sweat glands. J Invest Dermatol 1988;90:648–51.
18. Metze D, Kerssten A, Jurecka W, et al. Immunoglobulins coat microorganisms of skin surface: a comparative immunohistochemical and ultrastructural study of cutaneous and oral microbial symbionts. J Invest Dermatol 1991;96:439–45.
19. Puhvel SM, Warnick MA, Sternberg TH. Levels of antibody to Staphylococcus epidermidis in patients with acne vulgaris. Arch Dermatol 1965;92:88–90.
20. Puhvel SM, Warnick MA, Sternberg TH. Corynebacterium acnes. Presence of complement fixing antibodies to corynebacterium acnes in the sera of patients with acne vulgaris. Arch Dermatol 1966;93:364–6.
21. Asbee HR, Fruin A, Holland KT, et al. Humoral immunity to Malassezia furfur serovars A, B, and C in patients with pityriasis versicolor, seborrehic dermatitis and controls. Exp Dermatol 1994;3:227–33.
22. Asbee HR, Muir SR, Cunliffe WJ, et al. IgG subclasses specific to Staphylococcus epidermidis and Propionibacterium acnes in patients with acne vulgaris. Brit J Dermatol 1997;136:730–3.
23. Karvonen SL, Räsänen L, Cunliffe WJ, et al. Delayed hypersensitivity to Propionibacterium acnes in patients with severe nodular acne and acne fulminans. Dermatology 1994;189:344–9.
24. Kesavan S, Holland KT, Ingham E. The effects of lipid extraction on the immunomodulatory activity of Malassezia species in vitro. Med Mycol 2000;38:239–47.
25. Jappe U, Ingham E, Henwood J, et al. Propionibacterium acnes and inflammation in acne: P acnes has T-cell mitogenic activity. Brit J Dermatol 2002;146:202–6.
26. Elias PM. The skin barrier as an innate immune element. Semin Immunopathol 2007;29:3–14.
27. Bockmühl D, Jasoy C, Nieveler S, et al. Prebiotic cosmetics: an alternative to antibacterial products. IFSSC Mag 2006;9:1–5.
28. Harmesen HJ, Gibson GR, Elfferich P, et al. Comparison of viable ell counts and fluorescence in situ hybridization using specific rRNA-based probes for the quantification of human feel bacteria. FEMS Microbiol Lett 2000;183:125–9.
29. Holland KT, Bojar RA. Cosmetics. What is their influence on the skin microflora? Am J Clin Dermatol 2002;3:445–9.
30. de Jongh GJ, Zeuwen PL, Kucharekova M, et al. High expression levels of keratinocyte antimicrobial proteins in psoriasis compared with atopic dermatitis. J Invest Dermatol 2005;125:1163–73.
31. Kaila M, Isolauri E, Soppi E, et al. Enhancement of the circulating antibody secreting cell response in human diarrhea by a human Lactobacillus strain. Ped Res 1992;32:141–4.
32. Saavedra JM, Baumann NA, Oung I, et al. Feeding of Bifidobacterium bifidum and Streptococcus thermophilus to infants in hospital for prevention of diarrhoea and shedding of rotavirus. Lancet 1994;344:1046–9.

33. Sugita T, Togawa M. Efficacy of *Lactobacillus* preparation Biolactis powder in children with rotavirus enteritis. Jpn J Pediatr 1994;47:2755–62.

34. Shornikova AV, Casas I, Mykkänen H, et al. Bacteriotherapy with *Lactobacillus reuteri* in rotavirus gastroeneteritis. Ped Infect Dis J 1997;16:1103–7.

35. Link-Amster H, Rochat F, Saudan KY, et al. Modulation of a specific humoral immune response and changes in intestinal flora mediated through fermented milk intake. FEMS Immunol Med Microbiol 1994;10:55–63.

36. Isolauri E, Arvola T, Sütas Y, et al. Probiotics in the management of atopic eczema. Clin Exp Allergy 2000;30:1605–10.

37. Rosenfeldt V, Benfeldt E, Dam Nielsen S, et al. Effect of probiotic Lactobacillus strains in children with atopic eczema. J Allergy Clin Immunol 2003;111:389–95.

38. Viljnen M, Savilahti E, Haahtela, et al. Probiotics in the treatment of atopic eczema/dermatitis syndromein infants: a double-blind placebo-controlled trial. Allergy 2005;60:494–500.

39. Weston S, Halbert A, Rihmond P, et al. Effects of prebiotics on atopic dermatitis: a randomized controlled trial. Arch Dis Child 2005;90:892–7.

40. Abrahamson TR, Jakobsson T, Böttcher MF, et al. Probiotics in prevention of IgE-associated eczema: a double-blind, randomized, placebo-controlled trial. J Allerg Clin Immunol 2007;119:1174–80.

41. Pohjavuori E, Viljanen M, Korpela R, et al. *Lactobacillus* GG effect in increasing IFN-gamma production in infants with cow's milk allergy. J Allerg Clin Immunol 2004;114:131–6.

42. Lammers KM, Brigidi P, Vitali B, et al. Immunomodulatory effects of probiotic bacteria DNA: Il-1 and IL-10 response in human peripheral blood mononucelar cells. FEMS Immunol Med Microbiol 2003;38:165–72.

43. Prescott SL, Dunstan JA, Hale J, et al. Clinical effects of probiortics are associated with increased interferon-gamma responses in very young children with atopic dermatitis. Clin Exp Allerg 2005;35:1557–64.

44. Chapat L, Chemin K, Dubois B, et al. *Lactobacillus casei* reduces CD8+ T-cell-mediated skin inflammation. Eur J Immunol 2004;34:2520–8.

45. Gueniche A, Benyacoub J, Buetler TM, et al. Supplementation with oral probiotic bacteria maintains cutaneous immune homeostasis after UV exposure. Eur J Dermatol 2006;16:511–7.

46. Bouilly D, Jeannes C, Duteil L, et al. Probiotic and carotenoids: an innovative nutritional approach to help skin against sun damage. J Dermatol Sci, in press.

47. Puch F, Samson-Villeger S, Guyonnet D, et al. The consumption of functional fermented milk containing borage oil, green tea and vitamin E enhances skin barrier function. Exp Dermatol 2008;7:668–74.

48. Ouvehand AC, Batsman A, Salminen S. Probiotics of the skin: a new area of potential application? Lett Appl Microbiol 2003;36:327–31.

49. Gueniche A, Cathelineau AC, Bastien P, et al. *Vitreoscilla filiformis* biomass improves seborrheic dermatitis. JEADV 2007;17:1468–9.

50. Gueniche A, Hennino A, Goujon C, et al. Improvement of atoic dermatitzis skin symptoms by *Vitreoscilla filiformis* bacterial extract. EJD 2006;16:380–4.

Dermal Substitutes Do Well on Dura: Comparison of Split Skin Grafting +/− Artificial Dermis for Reconstruction of Full-thickness Calvarial Defects

R.A.J. Wain*, S.H.A. Shah, K. Senarath-Yapa,
J.K.G. Laitung

KEYWORDS

• Artificial dermis • Full thickness calvarial defects • Dura

The successful use of artificial dermal substitute has been well reported in the management and reconstruction of burns, and is becoming more common in general reconstruction and after oncological resection.[1] Studies have documented the use of artificial dermis for partial and full-thickness soft tissue scalp defects,[2] and one institution has described the use of Integra Bilayer Matrix Wound Dressing directly onto dura.[3]

We present the case of a 91-year-old lady with a history of four separate skin tumours of the scalp over the period of ten years, each of which underwent excision and differing methods of reconstruction. Two of these tumours necessitated full-thickness calvarial excision and resurfacing with either split skin grafting alone, or with split skin grafting and dermal substitute. We have found that artificial dermis along with split-thickness skin grafting provides an excellent option for closure of full-thickness calvarial defects. It offers an extra layer for dural protection and gives a better cosmetic result, whilst avoiding the invasive nature and prolonged recovery of other techniques.

CASE REPORT

A 91-year-old lady presented with a seven-month history of recurrent basal cell carcinoma (BCC) on the vertex of the scalp following excision some years previously. This patient had a history of three other skin tumours of the scalp, all of which required operative treatment and reconstruction over the last ten years.

The first tumour, approximately ten years ago, was a noninvasive BCC of the left frontal scalp. This was completely excised and the area resurfaced successfully using a split skin graft. The second tumour was an adherent, locally invasive squamous cell carcinoma (SCC) of the right frontal scalp which was excised along with the outer table

This article originally published in *Journal of Plastic, Reconstructive & Aesthetic Surgery (2010) 63, e826–e828,* *Elsevier.*
Conflicts of interest: None.
Funding: None.
Department of Plastic & Reconstructive Surgery, Royal Preston Hospital, Preston, Lancashire, UK
* Corresponding author.
E-mail address: richwain@doctors.org.uk

Clin Plastic Surg 39 (2012) 65–67
doi:10.1016/j.cps.2011.09.010

of calvarium. The defect was covered with a split skin graft directly to the inner calvarial table with good results.

Five years ago, in 2005, the patient underwent extensive surgery for a further infiltrative SCC on the right parietal scalp with bony involvement. The tumour was excised along with the full-thickness of the calvarium and closed using a split-thickness skin graft directly on to dura. The procedure pre-dated the introduction of artificial dermis in onco-logical reconstruction, and the presence of a skin graft and scarring from prior scalp surgery meant that local flap reconstruction was not practical.

Physical examination revealed a nodular cuta-neous lesion approximately 4 × 4 cm with irregular edges, crusting and telangectasia on the vertex of the scalp, to the left of mid-line. There was also a 5 × 5 cm discoid defect to the right of mid-line from the earlier SCC excision and reconstruction, and two further defects over the frontal region from previous surgery (**Fig. 1**). Tissue biopsy of the left-sided parietal lesion confirmed the presence of recurrent BCC and a cranial bone biopsy deep to the lesion revealed extensive bony infiltration

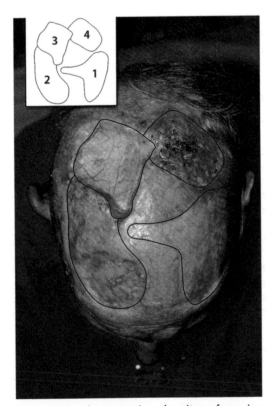

Fig. 1. Image demonstrating the sites of previous surgery and the current lesion. (1) Split skin graft onto scalp subcutaneous tissues; (2) Split skin graft to inner calvarial table; (3) Split skin graft to dura; (4) Site of Recurrent BCC.

with tumour penetrating almost the full thickness of the calvarium. A computed tomography (CT) head scan was performed which demonstrated the previous calvarial defect and showed no evi-dence of intracranial contrast-enhancing lesions.

Previous surgical procedures rendered local flap reconstruction impossible and, as the patient was frail, wheelchair bound, and had a past medical history of cardiovascular disease, invasive recon-structive techniques using free or pedicled flaps were not considered appropriate.

The patient underwent excision of the recurrent BCC including the involved cranial vault leaving an intact layer of dura exposed and a defect measuring 5 × 5 cm. In order to provide adequate oncological clearance, a larger area of scalp tissue was excised including the periosteum. The whole defect was thoroughly cleaned using iodine based solution and covered with Integra (Integra Dermal Reg-eneration Template, Integra LifeSciences Corp., Plainsboro, NJ, USA) which was sutured in place (**Fig. 2**A). Wound check at seven days showed 100% take of the Integra over the previously exposed dura. The defect was covered using a split-thickness skin graft at twenty-one days, and the dural wound was fully healed at eight weeks follow-up. The calvarial defect devoid of periosteum granulated well and healed by secondary intention. A direct comparison of the two healed dural wounds shows a much thicker and healthier result on the patient's left (graft + artificial dermis) in contrast to the thin, pale result on the patient's right with visible dural vasculature (graft alone) (see **Fig. 2**B).

DISCUSSION

Large, full-thickness skull defects present a series of significant challenges for both the patient and surgeon. For the patient this can involve multiple, prolonged operations with associated physical and emotional stresses, and of course the likeli-hood of a notable cosmetic defect. For the sur-geon, reconstructive techniques such as local flaps, bone grafts and free-tissue transfer are considered, but not always suitable for the patient group due to pre-existing co-morbidities, previous radiation therapy, distorted anatomy secondary to prior surgery, or ongoing bacterial contamination.

For the closure of large scalp and forehead wounds, many plastic & reconstructive surgeons choose free-tissue transfer due to the resilient blood supply and ability to shape and inset tissue to fit the defect.[4] Free flaps are durable, versatile and are available from a variety of anatomical sites, however the surgery is complex, time-consuming and patients require care in a specialist unit postoperatively.

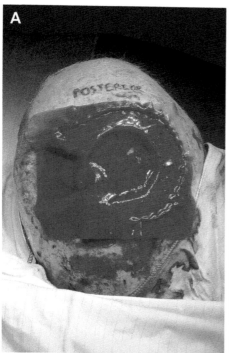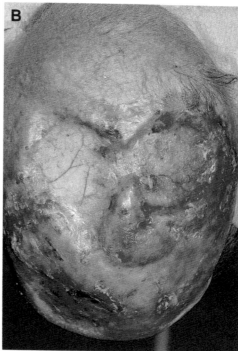

Fig. 2. (*A*) Artificial dermis sutured into place covering the full thickness calvarial defect. (*B*) Eight weeks post split skin grafting onto artificial dermis demonstrating the fuller and more substantial result on the patient's left, compared to skin grafting alone on the patient's right.

Other techniques for reconstruction of scalp defects include healing by secondary intention, skin grafting, tissue expansion, and local and regional flaps. Details of these methods are described in full by Seitz & Gottlieb.[4]

Due to our patient's previous scalp surgery, underlying medical condition, age, and general poor health, the options of free-tissue transfer or local flap cover were deemed unsuitable. In addition, the size of the defect and presence of exposed dura and calvarium left few remaining existing reconstructive solutions. The use of artificial dermis in burns reconstruction is well established[5] and is increasing in the treatment of oncological defects.[1,2] Integra Bilayer Matrix Wound Dressing in conjunction with topical negative pressure therapy and a split-thickness skin graft has been described once on a full-thickness calvarial defect.[3] We successfully used a similar technique in our patient with Integra Dermal Regeneration Template and split-thickness skin grafting without topical negative pressure therapy.

Our patient clearly demonstrates the different results of split skin grafting to cover dura with and without the use of artificial dermis. The most notable advantage of dermal substitute is the fuller and more substantial cover it provides when compared to simply split-thickness skin grafting. In circumstances where existing reconstructive methods are not suitable, artificial dermis coupled with split-thickness skin grafting can provide adequate tissue coverage and is preferable to skin grafting alone.

REFERENCES

1. Dantzer E, Braye FM. Reconstructive surgery using an artificial dermis (Integra): results with 39 grafts. Br J Plast Surg 2001;54:659–64.
2. Komorowska-Timek E, Gabriel A, Bennett DC, et al. Artificial dermis as an alternative for coverage of complex scalp defects following excision of malignant tumors. Plast Reconstr Surg 2005;115:1010–7.
3. Momoh AO, Lypka MA, Echo A, et al. Reconstruction of full-thickness calvarial defect: a role for artificial dermis. Ann Plast Surg 2009;62:656–9.
4. Seitz IA, Gottlieb LJ. Reconstruction of scalp and forehead defects. Clin Plast Surg 2009;36:355–77.
5. Heimbach D, Luterman A, Burke J, et al. Artificial dermis for major burns: a multicenter randomized clinical trial. Ann Surg 1988;208:313–20.

Management of Wounds with Exposed Bone Structures using an Artificial Dermis and Skin Grafting Technique

Xin Chen*, Hui Chen, Guoan Zhang

KEYWORDS

- Artificial dermis • Exposed bone • Non-healing wound

Problems associated with a non-healing wound are frequently noted in individuals with mechanical trauma and burns, pressure ulcers and diabetic illness. The task of managing such a wound, especially in instances with bony exposure, is clinically challenging, if not difficult.

Most treatment approaches involve conservative treatment and surgery. Currently, surgical treatment often uses local or distal skin flaps, muscle flaps or myocutaneous flaps to repair defects.[1]

The most simplistic approach in managing a wound that could not be closed primarily is to use a piece of skin graft for coverage. Although a skin flap mobilised from the area adjacent or from a distant site has been advocated to manage a wound with vital structures exposed, that is, bone, vessels and nerves, the techniques in practice are often plagued with problems such as paucity of flap donor sites. The magnitude of morbidities associated with these procedures further precludes their use.

Artificial dermis, with its silicone membrane, collagen–sponge bilayer structure, was the first tissue-engineered skin replacement that could be successfully used in clinical situations. Artificial dermis is mainly used to repair skin and soft tissue defects; it has also been used to successfully repair wounds with partial tendon exposure even with exposed bone wound.[2,3]

A regimen of wound management that includes the initial coverage of a newly freshened wound with an artificial dermis and grafting of the resultant wound with a piece of autologous partial-thickness skin graft was tried at our hospital in 17 wounds in 15 patients. The experience gained from managing this group of patients formed the basis of this article.

This article originally published in *Journal of Plastic, Reconstructive & Aesthetic Surgery (2010) 63, e512–e518*, Elsevier.

Conflict of interest: None of the authors has any commercial associations that might pose or create a conflict of interest with information presented in this article. Such associations include consultancies, stock ownership or other equity interests, patent licencing arrangements, and payments for conducting or publicising a study described in this article. The study protocol was approved by the Ethics Committee of the Beijing University Health Science Centre and conforms to the World Medical Association Declaration of Helsinki (June 1964).

Funding: There is no funding in any part of this clinical observation. No intramural or extramural funding supported any aspect of this work.

Department of Burns, Beijing Jishuitan Hospital, Beijing 100035, P.R. China

* Corresponding author.

E-mail addresses: xchin@sohu.com; xchin@vip.sina.com

doi:10.1016/j.cps.2011.09.011

Table 1
Summary of patient clinical characteristics

Patient	Age (y)	Gender	History Summary	Bone-exposed Part and Size	Wound Infection	Surgical Bed	Interval Between Surgeries (days)	Outcome	Follow-up Period (months)
1	72	Female	After steel plate internal fixation of right lateral malleolus fracture, the steel plate was exposed for 6 weeks. Patient had a >10-y history of diabetes.	Right lateral malleolus, 2 cm × 5 cm, exposed wound	Yes	Bone	20	Healed	18
2	43	Male	Left distal tibial open fractures with exposed ankle joint for 9 weeks.	Left distal tibial, 2 cm × 2.5 cm, exposed wound	Yes	Bone and exposed joint	Infected	Failed	18
3	39	Male	Wheel crush injury to the right leg. Severe skin abrasion and muscle laceration; tibia partially exposed for 2 weeks.	Right proximal tibia, 3 cm × 5 cm, exposed wound	Yes	Bone	16	Healed	12
4	34	Female	Right foot dorsum burn scar ulceration with exposed bone, 15-y history of repeated ulcerations.	Right foot dorsum metatarsals, 2 cm × 2.5 cm, exposed wound	· No	Bone	16	Healed	11
5	21	Male	Widespread skin and soft tissue necrosis after anhydrous ethanol injection for right leg lymphocele, 6-wk history.	Right proximal tibia, 3 cm × 18 cm, exposed wound	Yes	Bone	28 (First implantation) 15 (Second implantation)	Healed	10
6	33	Male	Right distal tibial and fibular open fractures, 38 days after external frame fixation.	Right tibia 3 cm × 5 cm, exposed wound, exposure of fracture ends	Yes	Bone	28	Healed	8
7	6	Male	Wheel crush injury to the right leg. Femur and tibia fracture, severe skin abrasion and necrosis; tibia partially exposed for 19 days.	Right tibia 1.5 cm × 3 cm, exposed wound	Yes	Bone and periosteum	15	Healed	5

No.	Age	Sex	History	Wound		Exposed tissue	Days	Outcome	Follow-up
8	30	Female	Wheel crush injury to the right lower leg and foot. Severe skin abrasion and muscle laceration; tibia, 5th dorsum metatarsal and calcaneus partially exposed for 26 days.	Right tibia 1 cm × 3 cm; Right 5th dorsum metatarsal 0.8 cm × 1 cm; Right calcaneus 3 cm × 3.5 cm, exposed wound	Yes	Bone and periosteum	14 14 Infected	Healed Healed Failed	8
9	28	Male	High voltage electronic burn injury to left foot, calcaneus and achilles tendon exposed for 6 weeks.	Left calcaneus 2 cm × 2.5 cm, exposed wound	Yes	Bone and periosteum	24	Healed	4
10	39	Male	Chemical burn to lower legs and feet; dorsum metatarsals and achilles tendon partially exposed for 9 weeks.	Left first dorsum metatarsal, 1 cm × 2 cm, exposed wound	Yes	Bone	21	Healed	2
11	36	Male	Crush injury to lower extremity; right thigh amputation; Severe skin avulsion to left lower leg; tibia partially exposed for 19 days.	Left tibia anterior part 3.5 cm × 22 cm, exposed wound	Yes	Bone	21	Healed	6
12	72	Female	Chronic ulcer to right knee with tibial tubercle exposed for 2 years.	Right tibial tubercle 1.5 cm × 1.5 cm exposed wound	No	Bone and periosteum	18	Healed	2
13	38	Male	Traffic accident crush to the right leg, excision of external malleolus after infection, chronic ulcer on external malleolus for 3 years, deep vein thrombosis	Right distal fibula 2.5 cm × 1.5 cm exposed wound	Yes	Bone and periosteum	20	Healed	1
14	43	Male	Chronic ulcer on left medial malleolus for 17 years.	Left medial malleolus 1.5 cm × 1.5 cm exposed wound	Yes	Bone and periosteum	14	Healed	1
15	29	Male	High voltage electronic burn injury to right leg and foot for two days.	Left tibia anterior part 3.8 cm × 12 cm, exposed wound	No	Bone and periosteum	21 (First implantation) 21 (Second implantation)	Healed	1

CLINICAL MATERIALS AND METHODS
Patient Materials

A total of 15 inpatients were treated during 2.5 years. There were 11 men and four women. While the youngest was 6 years, the oldest was 72 years, with a mean age of 38.14 ± 17.29 years. As noted in the **Table 1**, all wounds were located in the lower extremities and all had the underlying bony structures exposed **Fig. 1**. Mechanical trauma noted in 10 patients was the most common cause of the wounds while chemical burns in two and electrical burns in one were the causes. Breakdown of an old burn scar was the cause in the other patient.

Methods of Management

In every case, reconstruction was carried out in the same two-stage process. In the first stage, surgical debridement was carried out in all instances, in addition to removal of devitalised tissues; the bony surface was abraded lightly in instances without periosteal coverage **Fig. 1B**. After haemostasis was achieved, the wound was then carefully cleansed and disinfected with

povidone–iodine solution. In patient 1 who suffered from right lateral malleolus fracture fixed with a steel plate, the exposed metal work was first removed. A freshly treated wound, with its bacterial content ascertained, was covered with an artificial dermal template (Pelnac artificial dermis; Gunze Co., Ltd., Kyoto, Japan). The template is a bilayer xenographic dermal substitute composed of an atelocollagen matrix layer, which promotes dermal regeneration, and a semipermeable silicone layer, which functions as a temporary epidermis.[4–6] The size of the artificial dermis used, although depending upon the size of the wound, was larger than the actual bone-exposed wound size. The artificial dermis was anchored tightly by suturing or stapling along the wound edges. A nanometre silver antimicrobial dressing (SKNM, Seek Nano Medical Technology Co., Ltd., Nanjing, P.R.China) was also applied to cover the grafts with moderate pressure. The dressings were changed every 2–3 days and sutures or staples were removed 7 days after surgery. Fluid accumulated beneath the dermal template was drained by making a stab incision to the dermal template. Antibiotics covering

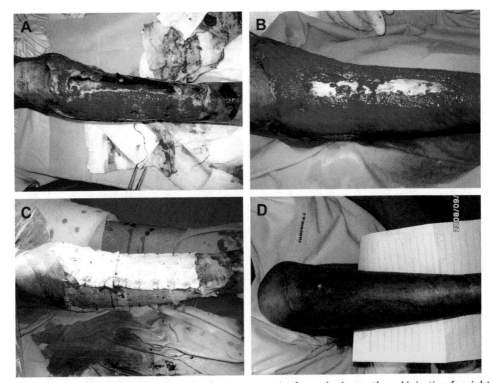

Fig. 1. (A) Patient 5 with widespread skin and soft tissue necrosis after anhydrous ethanol injection for right foreleg lymphocele 6 weeks after the injury, exposure of the tibia was 3 cm × 18 cm. (B) The wound was surgically debrided and the bony surface abraded. (C) The bony surface was covered with an artificial dermis while pieces of partial thickness skin graft were used to cover the remaining wound. (D) The appearance of reconstructed area one year later.

mostly the Gram-positive variants were used intravenously in all patients about 3–5 days after operation. Although the time elapsed varied, the wound would become sufficiently vascularised to accept a piece of an autologous partial-thickness skin graft in 2–4 weeks. During the second and final stages, the silicone layer was removed and the wound base was lightly abraded to determine the adequacy of revascularisation; light blood seepage is usually observed in a matured wound bed. The resultant wound was replaced with a thin split-thickness skin graft with its thickness varying between 8/1000th of an inch to 12/1000th of an inch. The grafted wound was managed in the usual manner: the graft was anchored to the wound base with sutures or staples and covered with a piece of petrolatum gauze impregnated with antibiotic ointment. A light compression dressing was used to protect the grafted area. The wound was uncovered 4–5 days later to ascertain the 'take' of skin graft **Fig. 1C**. The patient was observed for the next 6–12 months to ensure proper recovery from the procedure and the original injuries **Fig. 1D**.

FINDINGS AND RESULTS

As noted in the **Table 1**, there were 17 wounds treated in 15 patients. The size of the smallest wound was about 1 cm^2 while the largest was measured to be 22×4 cm^2. Although the periosteal covering was absent in 11 wounds, all wounds were managed in an identical manner. The foreleg wound with exposed bony tibia was the most common site while the ankle was involved in five instances.

The days needed to vascularise the dermal matrix, as expected, varied with wound size; it took 14 days for a small wound while a 3×18 cm wound took 4 weeks to complete. Wound coverage failed in two instances, thus requiring additional procedures. Infection was noted to be the factor responsible for the failure.

With an exception of repeat operation required in two patients, the morbidities associated with the procedures were nil. The structural integrity of grafted area in all instances was noted to be satisfactory; neither skin breakdown nor scar hypertrophy was observed.

FOLLOW-UP

On subsequent follow-up visits, all grafts on the artificial dermis showed satisfactory coverage without any complications such as breakdown, blister and chronic ulcer; even skin wrinkling of the grafts on the exposed bone were observed in several long follow-up cases; it demonstrated the pliability and stability of the grafts. In cases 1, 6 and 7 as well, the fractures healed well; further operations were needed to remove the orthopaedic fixtures. In addition, no significant hypertrophic scarring was observed at donor sites.

DISCUSSION

Artificial dermis, with its silicone membrane and collagen–sponge bilayer structure, has been widely used for coverage of full-thickness skin defect wounds with a simple STSG surgery on a well-vascularised wound bed. It is common surgical knowledge that autogenous or artificial skin grafts can take well on a wound bed with rich blood supply. However, the exposed bone wound often exhibited poor blood circulation, especially in exposed bone wound with periosteal defect. In this article, we describe our successful experience using artificial dermis to repair exposed open wounds in 15 patients who suffered from exposed bone wounds with periosteal defect in the lower extremity; this attempt had excellent outcomes.

The regimen of covering an open wound begins from the simplest technique of primary closure to the most complicated approach of using a microsurgical approach to transfer a compositae skin flap from a distant site. A chronically non-healing, especially in instances with exposed bony structures underneath, renders most of the conventional approaches in wound coverage not feasible. The use of a compositae tissue transfer technique, though preferred, may not be possible because of paucity of graft donor site and/or poor physical status.

An artificial dermis Integra, invented and its use advocated by Burke and Yannas initially in 1980,[4,5] was thought to be effective in covering an open wound as the artificial dermis could function as a dermal template. Pelnac artificial dermis is also a kind of a bilayer structured dermal substitute similar to Integra, but different in the origin of collagen and some biological characteristics (**Fig. 2**).[6–8] Until now, the artificial dermis had been widely used in repairing skin and soft-tissue defects. Ingrowth of capillaries, however, is said to be very difficult in a devitalised area (i.e., bony structures devoid of periosteal covering).

The periosteum plays a critical role not only in autogenous but also in artificial skin grafting on exposed bone wound bed. As shown in animals by Koga and his associates,[9] the periosteum is an essential tissue component of a wound bed with an exposed bone requiring skin grafting. The 'take' of a piece of partial-thickness skin graft

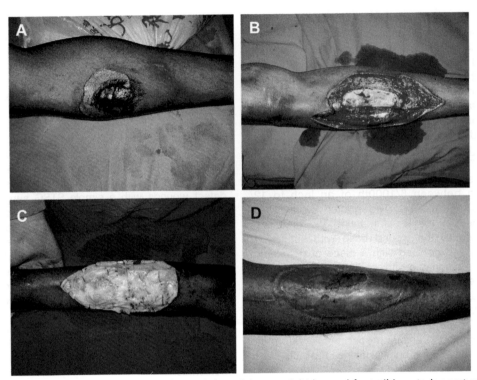

Fig. 2. (*A*) Patient 15 with high voltage electronic burn injury to right leg and foot, tibia anterior part partially exposed. (*B*) After 2 days of injury, a debridement and bone abrading was performed, the wound bed with exposed tibia in size of 3.8 cm × 12 cm was prepared for artificial dermis (Pelnac) implantation. (*C*) The wound was covered with an artificial dermis. (*D*) The appearance of reconstructed area one month later.

when applied to a bony surface without periosteal covering, in this regard, will be poor. The neo-vascularisation processes induced by decorticating the bone or drilling multiple holes into the medullary cavity, for instance, are unreliable and the extent of vascularised bed growth is unpredictable.

A complete co-aptation of a dermal template and a wound bed is essential for capillary ingrowth. The process of capillary bud invasion into the dermal matrix occurs from the base as well as from the wound periphery.[9] In an avascular bed, exemplified by bony structures devoid of periosteum, vascularisation of dermal template matrices would be initiated from the periphery. As noted in our patients, the vascularisation processes were prolonged. The effectiveness of decortication and cortical drilling to augment dermal template vascularisation was not clear from our observation.

Wound infection in the artificial dermis graft is still the main reason for failure as a result of the artificial dermis transplanted to bone-exposed wound; its survival will need a longer time. Preoperatively, the wound was treated and dressed by routine methods. Some patients underwent

systemic and local antibiotic treatment before-hand to control wound infection and inflammation until the wound was clean with no obvious remaining necrotic soft tissue. Intra-operatively, after thorough debridement, the wound site should be wet-compressed with povidone–iodine solution for about 5–10 min. It can effectively reduce wound infection. As a routine method, we use antimicrobials intravenously about 3–5 days after operation. In our study, there were only two cases of failure due to infection.

The conventional approach in covering a wound with exposed bone, specifically in the lower extremity, includes local flap technique, cross leg flap technique and distant flap technique via a microsurgical approach. The use of these techniques, in practice, is frequently barred by the magnitude of tissue defect and/or paucity of donor site. A staged approach using a dermal template and skin graft, however, definitely possesses effectiveness in wound management.

Although an artificial dermis, as shown by our patients as well as others,[10,11] is a useful template to fabricate a wound bed over pre-existing structures to support a piece of skin graft or a skin flap, the technique is technically time consuming. Various techniques to induce, enhance or 'encourage' the processes of neo-vascularisation in artificial dermis implanted have been described.[12,13] As shown by Jeschke and his associates, the combined use of fibrin glue and negative pressure therapy to an Integra-grafted area may reduce the time interval required for matrix vascularisation.[14] Further study is necessary to ascertain the technical manoeuvre to facilitate vascularisation processes in a larger group of patients. Nonetheless, the regimen is effective and it should be considered as an alternative mode of treatment when the use of other modalities is not possible.

SUMMARY

A staged approach in managing a non-healing wound, specifically in the lower extremity, using an artificial dermis and later, a piece of skin graft is effective, especially in instances where bony structures are exposed. The morbidities are low.

REFERENCES

1. Talbot SG, Pribaz JJ, Lee BT. A review of local and regional flaps for distal leg reconstruction. J Reconstr Microsurg 2009. [Epub ahead of print].
2. Joseph Molnar A, Anthony DeFranzo J, Hadaegh Anoush. Acceleration of integra incorporation in complex tissue defects with subatmospheric pressure. Plast Reconstr Surg 2004;113:1339–46.
3. Lee Lily F, Porch Juliet V, William Spenler C. Integra in lower extremity reconstruction after burn injury. Plast Reconstr Surg 2008;121:1256–62.
4. Yannas IV, Burke JF. Design of an artificial skin. I. Basic design principles. J Biomed Mater Res 1980;14:65–81.
5. Burke JF, Yannas IV, Quinby WC Jr, et al. Successful use of a physiologically acceptable artificial skin in the treatment of extensive burn injury. Ann Surg 1981;194:413–28.
6. Suzuki S, Matsuda K, Isshiki N, et al. Clinical evaluation of a new bilayer 'artificial skin' composed of collagen sponge and silicone layer. Br J Plast Surg 1990;43:47–54.
7. Suzuki S, Matsuda K, Maruguchi T, et al. Further applications of 'bilayer artificial skin'. Br J Plast Surg 1995;48:222–9.
8. Suzuki S, Kawai K, Ashoori F, et al. Long-term follow-up study of artificial dermis composed of outer silicone layer and inner collagen sponge. Br J Plast Surg 2000;53:659–66.
9. Koga Y, Komuro Y, Yamato M, et al. Recovery course of full-thickness skin defects with exposed bone: an evaluation by a quantitative examination of new blood vessels. J Surg Res 2007;137:30–7.
10. Yeong EK, Huang HF, Chen YB, et al. The use of artificial dermis for reconstruction of full thickness scalp burn involving the calvaria. Burns 2006;32:375–9.
11. Komorowska-Timek E, Gabriel A, Bennett Della C, et al. Artificial dermis as an alternative for coverage of complex scalp defects following excision of malignant tumors. Plast Reconstr Surg 2005;115:1010–7.
12. Soejima K, Chen X, Nozaki M, et al. Novel application method of artificial dermis: one-step grafting procedure of artificial dermis and skin, rat experimental study. Burns 2006;32:312–8.
13. Chen X, Soejima K, Nozaki M. Influence of mixed grafting of vascular endothelial cells and fibroblasts on the angiogenesis of artificial dermis. Chinese Journal of Burns 2006;22:452–5.
14. Jeschke MG, Rose C, Angele P, et al. Development of new reconstructive techniques: use of integra in combination with fibrin glue and negative-pressure therapy for reconstruction of acute and chronic wounds. Plast Reconstr Surg 2004;113:525–30.

Management of Split Skin Graft Donor Sites–Results of a National Survey

P.M. Geary*, E. Tiernan

KEYWORDS

• Skin graft • Donor site • Dressing • Survey

We report the findings of a postal survey of consultant opinion carried out in the later part of 2006. A postal questionnaire (Appendix 1) was sent to all consultants and locum consultant plastic surgeons with NHS/government practice in the British Isles asking about their management of split skin graft (SSG) donor sites.

We are preparing a protocol for a prospective randomised study of donor-site dressings. In order to make the study meaningful to the greatest number of practitioners, we wished to use, as a control, the dressing which was most frequently used in Britain. There is a large volume of literature worldwide on the subject of donor-site dressings, but we were unable to find an evidence to indicate the range of dressings used by British plastic surgeons, or which dressing was used the most. As the choice of donor-site dressing may be influenced by various factors (eg, size, anatomical site, need for re-harvesting and method of harvest), the questionnaire enquired into all these variables.

MATERIALS AND METHODS

On 1 July 2006, all the consultants and locum consultant plastic surgeons in the British Isles were identified from the BAPS website. All 61 listed plastic surgery units were contacted by telephone to confirm current NHS/government practice, and 357 consultant plastic surgeons were identified practising within the British Isles at this time.

Questionnaires were marked with a serial number and sent with a covering letter. All consultants were notified 2 weeks prior to distribution of questionnaires by email, letter or telephone, giving a brief outline of the study, including contact details. Of the 357 questionnaires sent, 210 were returned. After 2 months, 147 non-responders were contacted again as before, followed by a second posting of the questionnaire. Of which, 72 were returned.

RESULTS

In total, 283 questionnaires were returned, of which four were blank. The 279 completed questionnaires represent a response rate of 78%. All regions of the British Isles were well represented, with a minimum response rate above 65%. The highest response rate was from the South West of England (90%).

Frequency of Use of SSG

Respondents were asked to identify their approximate frequency of use of SSG. Over half of respondents used SSG weekly, and 36 had a major burns practice (**Table 1**).

Q1: Which of the Following Sites Do You Use as SSG Donors?

Respondents were asked to identify the frequency with which they used different anatomical sites as

This article originally published in *Journal of Plastic, Reconstructive & Aesthetic Surgery (2009) 62, 1677–1683*, Elsevier.

Odstock Centre for Burns and Plastic Surgery, Salisbury District Hospital, Odstock, Salisbury, Wiltshire, SP2 8BJ, UK
* Corresponding author. Department of Plastic Surgery, Salisbury District Hospital, Odstock, Salisbury, Wiltshire, SP2 8BJ, UK.
E-mail address: pmgeary@hotmail.com

Table 1
Estimated frequency of SSG use

Use of SSG	Number of Respondents
Frequent (~1 per week)	148
Rare (~1 per month)	77
Major burns practice	36
Blank	18

skin-graft donors. Seven anatomical locations were specified: buttock, thigh, instep, upper arm, forearm, hypothenar eminence and scalp. Respondents were also asked to specify any other site used. Separate estimates were requested for the frequency of use in children and in adult patients.

Respondents were asked to indicate if they used a given site routinely, once a month, once in 6 months, once a year, rarely or never. Respondents with major burns practice indicated a more frequent use of instep (in adults), forearm and upper arm (in children) and scalp (in both adults and children) when compared to non-burns surgeons. These results are summarised in **Table 2**.

Many surgeons feel that certain anatomical sites are unsuitable for the harvest of SSGs. In this survey, each of the given anatomical sites (apart from the thigh in adult patients) was avoided by some respondents. Almost half (47%) the respondents said they never used buttock as a donor site in adults, and one-third (33%) never used the thigh in children. In general, respondents were more likely to avoid a particular site in a child compared with an adult. The numbers of respondents

avoiding particular anatomical sites in adults and children are shown in **Table 3**.

Q2: What Methods of SSG Harvest Do You Use and with What Range of Settings?

Respondents were asked to indicate their use of powered or hand dermatomes in harvesting SSGs. The air dermatome was most commonly used, with the hand knife a close second. Ten respondents reported using all four dermatome types. These results are summarised in **Table 4**.

The Zimmer™ dermatome was the most commonly used air-powered dermatome (74 respondents out of 82 who specified a type). A small number of respondents used Aesculap™, Padgett™, Micro-Aire™ or Stryker™ models.

The most commonly used hand knife was the Watson (74 respondents out of 95 who specified a type). Other variants of the Humby knife accounted for most of the remainder. A small number used Weck/Goulian or Silver's knife.

Dermatome Thickness Settings

Of 228 respondents using air-powered dermatome, 45 gave no choice of setting. Of the remaining 183, choice of setting was highly variable. Some respondents gave a single setting; others gave a range of settings (shown graphically in **Fig. 1**).

Hand Knife Thickness Settings

Of the 201 respondents using a hand knife, 124 indicated their preferred thickness settings, Furthermore, 51 set the knife by eye, 11 used a scalpel blade as a 'feeler gauge', 14 used the marker notches on the knife (varying from less than one notch to four notches). Twenty-nine gave descriptive terms (eg, 'medium', 'just right'). Others gave small numbers without units, settings

Table 2
Anatomical sites used 'routinely'. Responses expressed as a percentage of all respondents (n = 279) and burns respondents (n = 36)

Anatomical Site	Adult		Child	
	All N (%)	Burns N (%)	All N (%)	Burns N (%)
Thigh	253 (91)	35 (97)	147 (53)	27 (75)
Buttock	73 (26)	14 (39)	159 (57)	22 (61)
Instep	20 (7)	5 (14)	17 (6)	3 (8)
Forearm	15 (5)	3 (8)	6 (2)	3 (8)
Upper arm	49 (18)	7 (19)	13 (5)	5 (14)
Hypothenar eminence	36 (13)	5 (14)	14 (5)	1 (3)
Scalp	39 (14)	12 (33)	39 (14)	13 (36)

Table 3
The number of respondents who reported that they never use a given anatomical site in children and in adults

Anatomical Site	Adult (%)	Child (%)
Thigh	0 (0)	92 (33)
Buttock	131 (47)	62 (22)
Instep	194 (70)	219 (78)
Forearm	201 (72)	248 (89)
Upper arm	142 (51)	235 (84)
Hypothenar eminence	155 (56)	213 (76)
Scalp	150 (54)	169 (61)

Table 4		
Types of dermatome used		
Dermatome	N (%)	Exclusive Use N (%)
Air powered	228 (82)	56 (20)
Hand knife	201 (72)	19 (7)
Battery powered	52 (19)	3 (1)
Mains powered	37 (13)	12 (4)
All types	10 (4)	

in thousandths of an inch, or set thickness by touch. Seventy-seven gave no setting preference.

Q3: What Donor-Site Healing Time Do You Tell (Adult) Patients to Expect (Weeks)?

The expected time for healing of an adult SSG donor site ranged from 7 to 42 days based on 266 respondents. Of these, more than half indicated an expected healing time of 14 days. Some respondents gave a single time, others a range (shown graphically in **Fig. 2**).

Q4: Do You Routinely Use Overgrafting of Donor Sites in The Elderly?

Slightly less than two-thirds of respondents (62%) reported the use of overgrafting of donor sites in elderly patients, including some who did so only in selected cases. Slightly more than one-third (35%) did not overgraft (the remaining 3% did not respond to this question).

Q5: How Long Would You Dress an Unhealed Donor Site Before Grafting (Months: Minimum/Maximum)?

The intention of this question was to obtain an indication of the time period within which most re-grafting of unhealed donor sites normally takes place. Many respondents gave a range, but

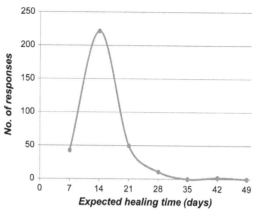

Fig. 2. Expected healing time of split skin graft donor site in adult patients. (Where a respondent gave a time range, this is represented as one response at each point within that range.)

some gave only a minimum time whilst others gave only a maximum time. Considering all of these responses together, the mean minimum time was 2 months; the mean maximum time was 4.2 months.

Q6: What Donor-Site Dressings Do You Use?

Presented with a choice of seven dressing types, respondents were asked to indicate which type was their dressing of choice, which ones they found acceptable and which they would only use in specific circumstances. They were also asked to indicate any other dressing material that they would use if it were available and any dressings they would avoid using.

The seven dressing types were: Alginate (eg, Kaltostat™), Plastic film (eg, Opsite™), Hydrocolloid (eg, Duoderm™), Adhesive fabric (eg, Mefix™), Paraffin gauze, Mepitel™ and Biobrane™.

SSG Donor-Site Dressings in Children

In **Figs. 3** and **4**, the horizontal bars indicate the number of respondents who reported using a given dressing type in children. Each bar is made up of three parts: those who use the dressing as their first choice (amber), those who felt its use was acceptable (blue) and those who would use it in certain circumstances (red).

SSG Donor-Site Dressings in Adults

Figs. 5 and **6** summarise the use of the seven dressing types in small (5 × 5 cm) and larger donor sites in adults. These charts show similar trends to those in children. Alginates are the most popular dressing in small and large donor sites, whether considering the first choice alone or overall use.

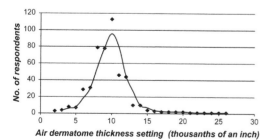

Fig. 1. Variation in the preferred air dermatome thickness settings (if a respondent indicated a range of thickness settings, eg, 8–12 thousandths of an inch, this is represented as one response for each of the thickness settings within that range).

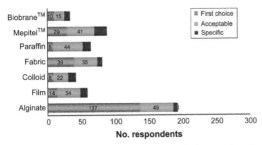

Fig. 3. Dressing preferences for small donor sites in children (≤5 × 5 cm).

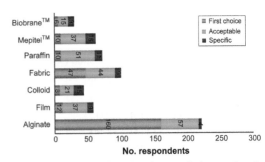

Fig. 5. Dressing preferences for small donor sites in adults (≤5 × 5 cm).

Fabric dressings are the second-most popular, both as first choice and overall.

Other dressing materials were identified by a small number of respondents (n). Lyofoam™ (n = 4), Mepilex border™ (n = 3) and Mepilex™ (n = 1), Aquacel™ (n = 1) and Aquacel AG™ (n = 1), Mepore™ (n = 1), Paracel™ (n = 1), Telfa™ (n = 7), Tisseel™ with Kaltostat™ (n = 1) and Tisseel™ with Opsite™ (n = 1).

Of the dressings that would be used if available, more respondents identified Biobrane™ than any other dressings, as shown in **Fig. 7**.

Each of the seven categories of dressing material were considered unsuitable for any donor site by approximately 10 respondents. The dressing materials most frequently avoided were paraffin gauze and plastic film (results summarised in **Fig. 8**).

Q7: In Choosing a Donor Dressing, What Order of Priority Do You Give These Criteria?

The majority of respondents gave a numerical order from 1 to 5. Some gave 'priority one' to several criteria. A small number gave non-numerical responses (tick or cross) to some or all of the alternatives. Where more than one criterion was marked as '1', all were scored as '1' and subsequent choices were re-numbered in numerical order. Non-numerical responses were scored equally as '1'. These five criteria were scored as

shown in **Table 5** (column totals do not add up to 279 as many respondents did not prioritise all options).

Based on these results, the most accepted order of priority is:

Pain>Healing time>Scar quality>Convenience>Cost

Q8: Do You Routinely Apply Local Anaesthetic for Postoperative Analgesia After GA Harvest?

In response to this question, 251 respondents (90%) reported routine use of local anaesthetic for postoperative pain relief and 28 respondents (10%) did not. The two most popular local anaesthetic agents were Bupivacaine (155) and Bupivacaine with Adrenaline (47). Other agents used included Laevobupivacaine ± Adrenaline (19/1), Lignocaine ± Adrenaline (4/1), Prilocaine ± Adrenaline (1/1), gels of Lignocaine (1) and Diclofenac (2) and peripheral nerve blocks, along with a wide range of combinations of two or more of the above.

Q9: How Do You Harvest SSG Under Local Anaesthesia?

Fifty-eight respondents (21%) reported harvest of skin graft using topical anaesthetic emulsion only. Eutectic mixture of local anaesthetics (EMLA™) was the most frequently used, but

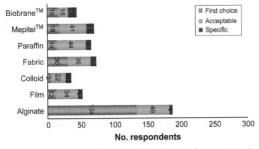

Fig. 4. Dressing preferences for larger donor sites in children (>5 × 5 cm).

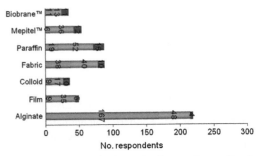

Fig. 6. Dressing preferences for larger donor sites in adults (>5 × 5 cm).

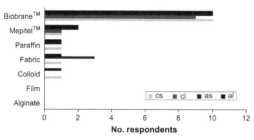

Fig. 7. Dressings that would be used if available. (Key: cs = child small, cl = child larger, as = adult small, al = adult larger.)

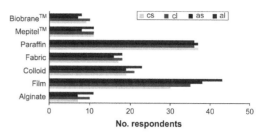

Fig. 8. Dressing to be avoided. (Key as for **Fig. 7.**)

more than half of respondents did not indicate their agent of choice.

DISCUSSION

In a Cochrane review of postal questionnaires,[1] three features were recognised as improving the response rate with an odds ratio (OR) of 2 or more.

> Interesting questions (OR = 2.44)
> Questionnaires sent by recorded delivery (OR = 2.21)
> Financial inducement (OR = 2.02)

A further three had a lesser positive influence with an OR greater than 1.5

> Short questionnaire (OR = 1.86)
> Pre-contact (OR = 1.54)
> Questionnaire in a brown envelope (OR = 1.52)

In order to maximise the response rate in this survey, respondents were pre-contacted, the questionnaire was on a single side of A4 and posted in a brown envelope.

In interpreting the results of this questionnaire, we have borne in mind that this is a survey of opinion and not based on verifiable results. Questions have been greatly simplified and do not inquire into reasons for choices (eg, how dressing choices are influenced by anatomical location of donor site).

Thigh and buttock are the most frequently used sites. All listed sites were used routinely by some respondents. The use of other anatomical sites was reported, especially in burns. In children, sites other than thigh and buttock are more rarely used than they are in adults.

The majority of respondents use a powered dermatome, but 73% of respondents use a hand knife in addition to other instruments and 7% of respondents use a hand knife exclusively. A recent discussion of medico-legal concerns regarding the use of a hand knife indicate that many plastic surgical consultants and trainees feel vulnerable to legal action in the event of causing a problem donor site by using a hand knife. However, in the opinion of the major defence organisations, this concern was unfounded. This was confirmed by communications with litigation departments in hospitals with a plastic surgery service who reported no such case on their records.[2]

Though the powered dermatome appears to take a more reliable skin graft in experienced hands, it is worth noting that a study of histological thickness of SSGs taken with a Zimmer™ dermatome showed a wide range of thickness.[3] This study concluded that there was no significant difference between the mean thickness of grafts taken with dermatome settings of 8, 9, 10 and 12 thousandths of an inch. There is uncertainty as to the effect of histological preparation methods on apparent graft thickness.

Advocates of the hand knife may argue that it is more portable and so more widely available, produces a non-linear margin to the donor-site scar (making it less noticeable than the straight-edged scar from a powered dermatome) and can be used to take a much wider graft, enabling larger defects to be covered with a single sheet. These considerations are reflected by the large number of respondents who still use a hand knife at times.

Expected healing times and planned re-grafting times were highly variable. There is however a clear indication that the majority of respondents advise patients to expect their donor site to be healed in 2 weeks, and re-grafting, if necessary, is likely to be carried out 2–4 months following the original operation.

Table 5
Number of respondents allocating priorities to dressing properties

Priority	1	2	3	4	5
Pain	**163**	50	31	8	1
Time	85	**96**	46	14	2
Scar	38	34	**73**	49	16
Convenience	45	29	58	**88**	15
Cost	90	8	3	9	**139**

Over-grafting of donor sites also has its proponents. There is no question that donor sites in elderly patients heal more quickly if over-grafted with highly meshed skin graft, compared with conventional dressings,[4,5] but the additional graft makes for a larger donor-site area.

The most frequent dressing of choice, in all four categories of donor site in this survey, was alginate. A small minority of respondents felt that alginates should be avoided. Adhesive fabric dressings were the second most frequent dressing of choice. They were the dressing of choice for approximately a quarter as many respondents as who chose alginates.

Of the suggested properties of donor-site dressings, pain was generally reported to be of prime importance. From existing prospective studies, alginates are associated with less pain than paraffin gauze,[6] but adhesive fabrics are associated with even less pain or discomfort when compared to alginates.[7,8] Hydrocellular foam is also associated with lesser pain than alginates.[9]

Healing time was the second most important dressing property. Alginates have been shown to result in reduced healing time when compared with paraffin gauze[6,10,16] and Mepitel™,[11] but an increased healing time compared with hydrocolloid dressing[12] and Scarlet Red.[13] Hydrocellular foam has been shown to speed healing in comparison to paraffin gauze.[14]

Scar quality was the third most important dressing property. Studies indicate better scar quality (and reduced bleeding), following dressing with alginate compared with paraffin gauze in paediatric scalp grafts.[15]

Of the dressings that would be used if available, Biobrane™ was the most frequently cited. Biobrane™ has undoubted value in the management of superficial burns, but its value as an SSG donor-site dressing is unproven. Two prospective studies of this dressing indicate that it results in less pain and discomfort than Scarlet Red[17] but is associated with a higher rate of infection.[17,18] Cost may be another factor despite this being the least important consideration in making a dressing choice. To dress a 5×5-cm donor site with Biobrane™ costs £37.40, compared with £1.83 for alginate, and 5 p for Mefix™.

There are clear incongruities between practice and published evidence. There are many published studies investigating dressings that are no longer available in the UK and many in which the control dressing is paraffin gauze, which is now rarely used, making the results difficult to interpret. A similar survey has been conducted before,[19] but there are no previously published British data, so it is not possible to comment on the

changes in practice. Some of the evidence points to adhesive fabrics being the best donor-site dressing, and their use is certainly greater now than it was 10 years ago. Only future study will show if its use continues to increase in the light of published evidence. At present, we feel that any future study of a new donor-site dressing should have the material which is currently the first choice for the majority of British plastic surgeons, namely Kaltostat™, as its control.

ACKNOWLEDGMENTS

The authors would like to thank the Salisbury Plastic Surgery Trust Fund for their generous financial support of this work.

REFERENCES

1. Edwards P, Roberts I, Clarke M, et al. Methods to increase response rates to postal questionnaires. Cochrane Database Syst Rev 2007;2:MR000008.
2. Tehrani H, Lindford A, Logan AM. Hand knife versus powered dermatome: current opinions, practices and evidence. Ann Plast Surg 2006;57:77–9.
3. Malpass KG, Snelling CFT, Tron V. Comparison of donor site healing under xeroform and jelonet dressings: unexpected findings. Plast Reconstr Surg 2003;112:430–9.
4. Ablaza VJ, Berlet AC, Manstein ME. An alternative for the split skin-graft donor site. Aesth Plast Surg 1997;21:207–9.
5. Converse JM, Robb-Smith AHT. The healing of surface cutaneous wounds: its analogy with the healing of superficial burns. Ann Surg 1944;120: 873–85.
6. Attwood AI. Calcium alginate dressing accelerates split skin graft donor site healing. Br J Plast Surg 1989;42:373–9.
7. Giele H, Tong A, Huddleston S. Adhesive retention dressings are more comfortable than alginate dressings on split skin graft donor sites – a randomised controlled trial. Ann R Coll Surg Engl 2001; 83:431–4.
8. Hormbrey E, Pandya A, Giele H. Adhesive retention dressings are more comfortable than alginate dressings on split skin graft donor sites. Br J Plast Surg 2003;56:498–503.
9. Vaingankar NV, Sylaidis P, Eagling V, et al. Comparison of hydrocellular foam and calcium alginate in the healing and comfort of split thickness skin-graft donor sites. J Wound Care 2001;10:289–91.
10. O'Donoghue JM, O'Sullivan ST, Beausang ES, et al. Calcium alginate dressings promote healing of split skin graft donor sites. Acta Chir Plast 1997;39:53–5.
11. O'Donoghue JM, O'Sullivan ST, O'Shaughnessy M, et al. Effects of a silicone-coated polyamide net

dressing and calcium alginate on the healing of split skin graft donor sites: a prospective randomised trial. Acta Chir Plast 2000;42:3–6.

12. Porter JM. A comparative investigation of re-epithelialisation of split skin graft donor areas after application of hydrocolloid and alginate dressings. Br J Plast Surg 1991;44:333–7.

13. Lawrence JE, Blake GB. A comparison of calcium alginate and scarlet red dressings in the healing of split thickness skin graft donor sites. Br J Plast Surg 1991;44:247–9.

14. Martini L, Reali UM, Borgognoni L, et al. Comparison of two dressings in the management of partial–thickness donor sites. J Wound Care 1999;8:457–60.

15. Pannier M, Martinot V, Castede JC, et al. Evaluation de l'efficacite et de la tolerance d'Algosteril (compresse d'alginate de calcium) versus Jelonet (gaze paraffinee) dans le traitement du site donneur de greffe dermo-epidermique du cuir chevelu. Resultats d'un essai pediatrique. Ann Chir Plast Esthet 2002;47:285–90.

16. Steenfos HH, Agren MS. A fibre free alginate dressing in the treatment of split thickness skin graft donor sites. J Eur Acad Dermatol Venereol 1998;11: 252–6.

17. Prasad JK, Feller I, Thompson PD. A prospective controlled trial of Biobrane versus Scarlet red on skin graft donor areas. J Burn Care and Rehab 1987;8:384–6.

18. Feldman DL, Rogers A, Karpinski RHS. A prospective trial comparing Biobrane, Duoderm and Xeroform for skin graft donor sites. Surg Gynecol Obstet 1991;173: 1–5.

19. Lyall PW, Sinclair SW. Australasian survey of split skin graft donor site dressings. Aust N Z J Surg 2000;70:114–6.

APPENDIX 1: THE QUESTIONNAIRE

Q1 - Which of the following sites do you use as SSG donors?

	Child	Adult
Buttock		
Thigh		
Instep		
Upper arm		
Forearm		
Hypothenar eminence		
Scalp		
Other (specify)		

Use of SSG	tick
Rare (~1/month)	
Frequent (~1/week)	
Major burns practice	

1	routinely
2	~ 1/ month
3	~ 1/ 6month
4	~1/yr
5	rarely
blank	never

Q2 - What methods of SSG harvest do you use and with what range of settings?

	Type	Setting Range
Hand Knife		
Air driven		
Battery driven		
Mains driven		

Q3 - What donor site healing time do you tell (adult) patients to expect? (wks)

Q4 - Do you routinely use overgrafting of donor sites in the elderly?

Q5 - How long would you dress an unhealed donor site before regrafting? (months)

Yes	No
min	
max	

Q6 - What SSG donor dressings do you use?

*("Small" = 5x5 cm or less)	Child		Adult	
	Small*	Large	Small*	Large
Alginate (e.g.Kaltostat,Sorbsan)				
Plastic film (e.g. Opsite, Tegaderm)				
Hydrocolloid (e.g. Duoderm)				
Adhesive fabric (e.g. Mefix, Hypafix)				
Paraffin gauze (e.g. Jelonet, Paranet)				
Mepitel				
Biobrane				
Other (1)				
Other (2)				

1	preferred
2	acceptable
3	in specific cases
4	avoid
5	would use if available
blank	no view

Q7 - In choosing a donor dressing, what order of priority do you give these criteria?

	Priority
Pain	
Healing time	
Scar quality	
Convenience	
Cost	
Other (specify)	

Q8 - Do you routinely apply Local Anaesthetic for postoperative analgesia after GA harvest?

Agent of choice	

Q9 - How do you harvest SSG under Local?

	agent used
Emulsion only	
Emulsion and infiltration	
Infiltration only	
Rarely take SSG under Local	

Skin: Histology and Physiology of Wound Healing

Eric A. Gantwerker, MS, MD[a], David B. Hom, MD[b],*

KEYWORDS

- Scarring • Scars • Facial • Wounds • Healing
- Skin histology

Key Points

1. Skin is composed of several layers that are essential to its function and response to injury: the epidermis, dermis, and hypodermis. Healing is a dynamic progression encompassing hemostasis, inflammation, proliferation, and remodeling

2. Pilosebaceous units are the source of all epithelial stem cells essential for reepithelialization and wound healing

3. Multiple extrinsic and intrinsic factors affect healing, specifically the effect of immune system modulation (medications and diseased states)

4. It is most optimal to wait at least 4–6 weeks after smoking cessation for elective surgical interventions

5. Keloids and hypertrophic scarring are a result of overabundant collagen production, and decrease collagen breakdown. Keloids are difficult to treat, due to their recurrent nature. It is important to identify individuals prone to keloid formation for surgical planning purposes

---

Self-Test Questions

The following questions are intended for the reader to self-test. The answers, with full background, are covered within this article.

The correct answers are provided at the conclusion of the article.

1. A 19-year-old woman is on isotretinoin (Accutane) for acne and has a facial acne scar that she wishes to be dermabraded. What do you counsel the patient about?
   a. She needs to be off the medication for 1 year to limit the risk of scarring
   b. She should continue the medication because the extra vitamin A will improve her healing
   c. You cannot resurface her acne scar because of the long-lasting effects of this medication
   d. Encourage 2 g of vitamin C daily for 2 weeks before the procedure

2. A 73-year-old insulin-dependent diabetic man with a serum glucose level of 300 mmol/L comes to your office for a rhytidectomy. How do you optimize your results?
   a. Refer to endocrinologist for tight diabetic control before surgery
   b. Decline the surgery because the risk of failure is increased
   c. Start the patient on vitamin E supplementation 2000 IE daily 2 weeks before surgery
   d. Double his insulin dose on the morning of his surgery

3. A 30-year-old man has a partial-thickness 4 × 4-cm abrasion on his right cheek. What should be the best treatment?

This article originally published in *Facial Plastic Surgery Clinics*, August 2011, 19:3.

Disclosures: There are no affiliations, conflicts of interest, or financial disclosures by either author.

[a] Department of Otolaryngology – Head and Neck Surgery, University of Cincinnati and Cincinnati Children's Hospital Medical Center, 231 Albert Sabin Way, Cincinnati, OH, USA

[b] Division of Facial Plastic and Reconstructive Surgery, Department of Otolaryngology – Head and Neck Surgery, University of Cincinnati and Cincinnati Children's Hospital Medical Center, 231 Albert Sabin Way, PO Box 670528, Cincinnati, OH 45267-0528, USA

* Corresponding author.

E-mail address: david.hom@uc.edu

Clin Plastic Surg 39 (2012) 85–97

doi:10.1016/j.cps.2011.09.005

a. Place a split-thickness skin graft
b. Place a full-thickness skin graft
c. Keep the wound bed moist with a moisture retentive ointment
d. Keep the wound dry to maximize reepithelialization.

4. A 50-year-old man sees you about a large wide scar on his neck. On inquiring, the patient states he had a lymph node removed last year and this scar has grown bigger than the cyst was. What do you counsel him about?
   a. That he most likely has a hypertrophic scar and that the likelihood is that this will not happen on further surgical procedures
   b. That this is a keloid and that with vitamin E ointments it should resolve
   c. That this is a hypertrophic scar that will completely go away with simple excision
   d. That this is a keloid and that multiple procedures along with steroid injections may be required to excise it, but still there is no guarantee it will be removed completely.

The study and treatment of wounds go back to Ancient Egypt. In Ancient Egypt the clean edges of wounds were brought together with tape or stitches and a piece of meat was placed on the wound for the first day. Salves such as honey and Matricaria oil were used. The antibacterial and antiseptic properties of these compounds were later elucidated. Honey was later found to have mild antibacterial effects in controlling *Pseudomonas* and methicillin-resistant *Staphylococcus aureus*.[1] Other wound dressings and salves have been used throughout history until the advent of germ theory, which revolutionized medicine and made a significant impact on surgery and wound care. Research in the last decade has focused on growth factors and cytokines that control the complex wound-healing cascade. Newer research has focused on modulating these signaling molecules to improve healing and prevent scarring.

Wound healing in this article focuses on:

- Basic histologic characteristics of skin
- Four phases of wound healing
- Brief overview of collagen matrices
- Extrinsic and intrinsic factors that disrupt wound healing
- Scarring and current classifications
- Basic principles of wound care and scar treatment.

Although each surgeon has his or her own techniques, some based on evidence and others based on preferences, there are certain tenets that most agree on. Here the authors cover some of the evidence supporting practices, but in the absence of definitive research their personal experience is relied upon.

The process of wound healing is a dynamic, complex interplay of cytokines, involving many different cell types. The skin has important immune and protective characteristics and has an amazing ability to heal, invariably with scarring. Scarring is quite variable and is based on many factors, dependent on patient characteristics and overall health (intrinsic) as well as the healing environment (extrinsic). All epithelial tissues in the body, except for bone, heal by scar formation rather than regeneration. The skin is not spared by this. It is important to identify wound-healing problems early to minimize scarring.

To understand the effects of injury and potential for scarring, one must first look at the layered histology and physiology of the largest organ in the body. The skin is separated into an epidermis, dermis, and hypodermis. The epidermis itself has 5 layers or strata from superficial to deep: corneum, lucidum, granulosum, spinosum, and basale (**Fig. 1**). The epidermis has variable thickness,

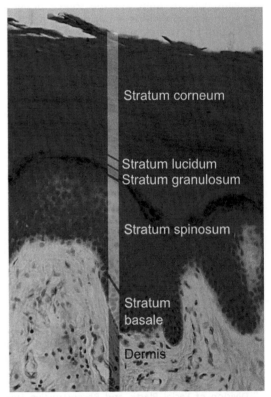

Fig. 1. Histologic section of the epidermis showing the 5 strata from superficial to deep: corneum, lucidum, granulosum, spinosum, and basale. (*Courtesy of* Mikael Haggstrom, Uppsala, Sweden; under GNU Free Documentation License. Available at: http://commons.wikimedia.org/wiki/File:Epidermal_layers.png.)

being thinnest on the eyelids and thickest on the palms and soles.[2,3] This thickness has implications in tissue healing and eventual scarring. The epidermal avascular layer receives its nutrients by diffusion through the dermal layer.

SKIN HISTOLOGY

Keratinocytes make up 95% of the epidermis, and the stratum basale is the source of all replicating keratinocytes. It is these keratinocytes in the basal layer that are primarily responsible for the epidermal response in wound healing.[4] As keratinocytes replicate they push older cells toward the surface, and these cells progressively lose their nucleus and take on a more flattened ovoid shape. This stratified squamous keratinized epithelium undergoes constant turnover, essentially regenerating fully every 48 days. The stratum basale sends down finger-like projections that interdigitate with similar structures reaching up from the dermis. This process forms the rete ridges that are often seen in cross section. Freshly healing wounds as well as skin grafts lack these rete ridges initially, which makes them susceptible to shear trauma early on.

The epidermis also contains essential appendages including hair follicles with associated sebaceous glands (pilosebaceous unit), eccrine sweat glands, and apocrine glands. The pilosebaceous unit, as well as rete ridges, contains epithelial stem cells that are able to regenerate and differentiate into basal keratinocytes and are essential to the reepithelialization process (**Fig. 2**). These stem cells are critical, as they are relatively undifferentiated, have a large proliferation potential, and have a high capacity for self-renewal.[5] Healing difficulties are seen when these stem cells are destroyed by insults such as burns and even iatrogenic sources such as dermabrasion. When dermabrasion or resurfacing is taken too deep it can destroy the apocrine glands and pilosebaceous unit, leading to improper healing and eventual scarring. Retinoid treatments such as isotretinoin (Accutane) cause atrophy of the sebaceous glands, which is the source of their effectiveness to treat acne. Isotretinoin leads to obvious problems with wound healing, directly

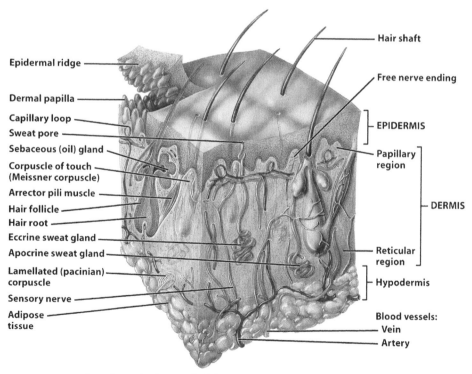

Sectional view of skin and subcutaneous layer

Figure 5-1a Anatomy and Physiology: From Science to Life
© 2006 John Wiley & Sons

Fig. 2. The many appendages of the epidermis and dermis. The pilosebaceous unit is the source of all stem cells essential to the reepithelialization process. (*Reprinted from* Jenkins GW, Tortora GJ, Kemniitz CP. Anatomy and physiology: from science to life. New York: J. Wiley and Sons; 2006. p. 148–71. Chapter: 5; with permission.)

reducing the cells needed for reepithelialization. Most surgeons would agree that patients should be off isotretinoin for at least 1 year prior to any surgical resurfacing procedure.[6]

The dermis is the next layer down, which receives the major blood supply for the skin and contains most of the dermal appendages of the skin including the apocrine glands, eccrine glands, and hair follicles. This layer itself is separated into a superficial or papillary dermis and the deeper reticular dermis. As a general rule, any damage that extends into this deeper reticular layer will invariably cause scarring and may require repair with full-thickness grafts or flaps to assure proper healing.

In general there are 4 overlapping phases of wound healing (**Fig. 3**):

1. Hemostasis
2. Inflammation
3. Proliferation
4. Maturation/remodeling.

Although these phases are separated for simplicity reasons they in fact overlap a great deal, and even different areas of wounds can be in different phases of healing. Any interruption in the natural cascade of healing can disrupt subsequent phases and can potentially result in abnormal healing, chronic wounds, and eventual scarring.[4]

Hemostasis

Hemostasis is the initial phase that occurs within seconds to minutes after the initial insult. Initially hemorrhage into the wound exposes platelets to the thrombogenic subendothelium. Platelets are integral to this phase and the entire healing pathway, as they not only serve to provide initial hemostasis but also release multiple cytokines, hormones, and chemokines to set off the remaining phases of healing. Vasoactive substances such as catecholamines and serotonin act via specialized receptors on the endothelium to cause vasoconstriction of the surrounding blood vessels. Smaller vessels are signaled to vasodilate to allow the influx of leukocytes, red blood cells, and plasma proteins. Platelets interact with the GpIIb-IIIa receptor on the collagen of the damaged subendothelium to become activated and form an initial clot. Activated platelets release their granules and ignite the extrinsic and intrinsic coagulation cascades. Fibrin polymerization helps form a mature clot and serves as scaffolding for the infiltrating cells (leukocytes, keratinocytes, and fibroblasts) that are key to subsequent phases of healing. Platelets release

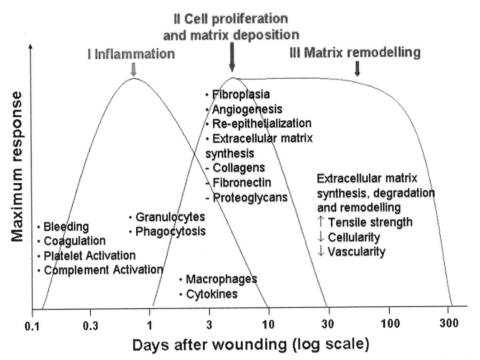

Fig. 3. Time scale of the 4 phases of healing and the many processes that occur at each phase of healing. Any disruption in these processes will ultimately delay healing and lead to scar formation. (*From* Enoch S, Price P. Worldwide Wounds. Available at: http://www.worldwidewounds.com/2004/august/Enoch/Pathophysiology-Of-Healing.html; with permission.)

a myriad of chemokines and cytokines to attract these inflammatory cells to the area. Within minutes, there is an influx of inflammatory cells (predominantly neutrophils and macrophages), leading to the next phase of healing.

Inflammation

The inflammatory phase is heralded by the influx of neutrophils, macrophages, and lymphocytes to the site of injury (**Fig. 4**). Neutrophils are the first leukocytes on site, arriving en masse within the first 24 hours. Neutrophils are soon followed by macrophages, which are attracted by the by-products of neutrophil apoptosis. Phagocytic cells such as macrophages and other lymphocytes appear in the wound to begin to clear debris and bacteria from the wound. These macrophages infiltrate at approximately 48 hours post injury and stay until the conclusion of the inflammatory phase. Macrophages have long been thought to be the key cell to the wound-healing process, and they seem to orchestrate the most important phases of healing. Although they are integral to proper healing, recent research has also looked at their role in improper healing and scarring. Studies of macrophage function have revealed that these key cells are intricate in reepithelialization, granulation tissue formation, angiogenesis, wound cytokine production, and wound contracture.[7] Inflammation is a necessary step of the healing process, and inhibition of this key phase (via anti-inflammatory medications) can result in improper healing. This phase of healing is important to combat infection.[8] If disrupted or prolonged (ie, longer than 3 weeks), this inflammation can lead to a chronic wound, impaired healing, and eventually more scarring. Important factors that can abnormally lengthen this phase of healing include high bacterial load (greater than 10^5 microorganisms per gram of tissue), repeated trauma, and persistent foreign material in the wound.[6] Once the wound has been debrided, the repair or proliferative phase begins.

Proliferation

The proliferative (repair) phase begins early on in the form of reepithelialization (**Fig. 5**). The repair phase also involves capillary budding and extracellular matrix production to fill in the defects left behind from debridement of the wound. Epithelialization is marked by the proliferation and influx of keratinocytes near the leading edge of the wound. As discussed previously, stem cells within the bulbs of the hair follicles and apocrine glands begin to differentiate into keratinocytes and repopulate the stratum basale, and also begin to migrate over the edge of the wound. Once they encounter the mesenchyme of the extracellular matrix (ECM), they attach near the inner wound edge and begin to lay down a new basement membrane. Following this, another row of keratinocytes migrates over the newly laid epithelial cells to fill in the defect. These cells migrate and digest the ECM using proteases until they are in physical contact and they stop migrating, signaled by contact inhibition from neighboring keratinocytes.[9] This reepithelialization protects the wound from infection and desiccation.

Deep wound healing

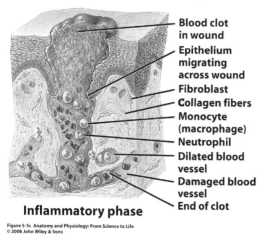

Blood clot in wound
Epithelium migrating across wound
Fibroblast
Collagen fibers
Monocyte (macrophage)
Neutrophil
Dilated blood vessel
Damaged blood vessel
End of clot

Inflammatory phase

Figure 5-5c Anatomy and Physiology: From Science to Life
© 2006 John Wiley & Sons

Fig. 4. The inflammatory phase heralded by the influx of neutrophils and macrophages into the wound. (*Reprinted from* Jenkins GW, Tortora GJ, Kemniitz CP. Anatomy and physiology: from science to life. New York: J. Wiley and Sons; 2006. p. 148–71. Chapter: 5; with permission.)

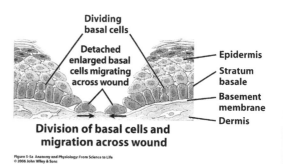

Dividing basal cells
Detached enlarged basal cells migrating across wound
Epidermis
Stratum basale
Basement membrane
Dermis

Division of basal cells and migration across wound

Figure 5-5a Anatomy and Physiology: From Science to Life
© 2006 John Wiley & Sons

Fig. 5. Reepithelialization takes place as keratinocytes differentiate from the stem cells in the basal stratum and migrate over the wound edge to fill in the defect. Migration stops, signaled by contact inhibition as the wound defect fills in. (*Reprinted from* Jenkins GW, Tortora GJ, Kemniitz CP. Anatomy and physiology: from science to life. New York: J. Wiley and Sons; 2006. p. 148–71. Chapter: 5; with permission.)

During this process a layer of uninfected exudates lies over the wound, which provides an important moisture layer and contains growth factors essential to healing. Any improper wound dressings that destroy this healthy layer will result in delayed healing. Underneath this reepithelialization process the ECM continues to be laid down. Wounds healing by secondary intention fill in with granulation tissue. Under the influence of vascular endothelial growth factor (VEGF), angiogenesis begins as the vessels begin to bud from the blood vessels surrounding the wound. Granulation tissue consists of these fibroblasts, new budding vessels, and immature collagen (collagen type III). Some fibroblasts will also begin to differentiate in this phase into myofibroblasts that have contractile function to bring gaping wound edges together.[8]

Angiogenesis/Maturation

Angiogenesis follows a typical pattern of sprouting, looping, and pruning signaled by a complex gradient of cytokines. These small and delicate sprouting vessels repopulate the dermis, and any trauma to this area will lead to destruction of these vessels and delayed healing. Shearing of these new vessels is often a problem in skin grafting, whereby the graft is solely supplied by initial imbibition for 24 hours followed by growth of these vessels into the tissue. It is the role of the bolster placed over these delicate graft sites to prevent hematoma that would limit diffusion of nutrients, but more importantly to prevent shearing of these delicate immature vessels. Bolsters are usually left on for 5 to 7 days to allow these vessels to become more robust and mature, and to resist these shearing forces. Angiogenesis is also a key process affected by primary versus secondary closures. Angiogenesis is greatly accelerated by primary closure, due to the proximity of the budding vessels. In healing through secondary intention, this process takes place through formation of the aforementioned granulation tissue induced by hypoxia, elevated lactate, and various growth factors. Healing by secondary intention involves epithelialization over this granulation and then extensive remodeling. Any medications that interfere with new blood vessel formation (ie, the antiangiogenic drug bevacizumab [Avastin]) can be detrimental to wound healing.

Remodeling

The remodeling phase begins as the provisional ECM and type III collagen is replaced with type I collagen and the remaining cell types of the previous phases undergo apoptosis (**Fig. 6**). With the laying down of type I collagen, the tensile

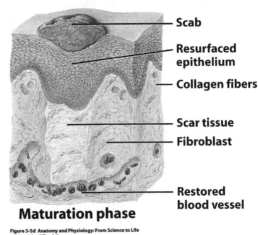

Deep wound healing

Scab

Resurfaced epithelium

Collagen fibers

Scar tissue

Fibroblast

Restored blood vessel

Maturation phase

Figure 5-5d Anatomy and Physiology: From Science to Life
© 2006 John Wiley & Sons

Fig. 6. The maturation phase is longest of the 4 phases and results in the final appearance of the wound. (*Reprinted from* Jenkins GW, Tortora GJ, Kemniitz CP. Anatomy and physiology: from science to life. New York: J. Wiley and Sons; 2006. p. 148–71. Chapter: 5; with permission.)

strength of the wound dramatically increases. Granulation tissue begins to involute and excess blood vessels retract. This phase lasts the longest and results in the final appearance of the wound following healing. A successful remodeling phase involves a delicate balance requiring synthesis more than lysis. Synthesis is greatly energy dependent, and any depletion of nutrients will push the balance toward lysis and affect the healing process. Excess fibrosis at this stage results in hypertrophic scarring (with the scar limited to the wound area) or keloid formation (with the scar extending beyond wound edge). The difficulty in treating both of these entities has targeted many research dollars on the prevention of scarring, and is discussed by Douglas Sidle, in detail in an article elsewhere in this issue.

Primary and Secondary Healing

It is important to discuss in brief the differences between primary and secondary healing. Primary healing is that which is seen in surgical wounds that involve uncomplicated healing of noninfected, well-approximated wounds (**Fig. 7**). These wounds follow the 4 phases of healing without abruption. Any disruptions in healing such as infection, dehiscence, hypoxia, or immune dysfunction will lead to a compromised wound that enters a stage of secondary healing.[10,11] If no intervention is undertaken, these wounds may become chronic wounds. Chronic wounds are out of the purview tumor, and calor" (pain, redness, growth, and heat).[10] Healing by secondary intention, as discussed previously, involves creation of granulation tissue and epithelialization over this healthy granulation tissue. Because angiogenesis and epithelialization takes longer in this setting, they are more prone to infection and poor healing. With proper care, healing by secondary intention may result in acceptable cosmesis on concave surfaces of the face.

Collagen in Wound Healing

Collagen is the single most abundant protein in mammals, and accounts for approximately 30% of our body's total protein content. Collagen and its triple helical structure have been studied for decades, and its structure was first described in the 1930s. Collagen is made from 3 alpha strands of left-handed helices that coil together to form the right-handed helix of a collagen fibril. These fibrils cross-link together via hydrogen bonds to form fibers. The molecular structure of collagen, as for all proteins, is essentially amino acids. The regular arrangement of collagen amino acids (Gly-Pro-X) provides for a great amount of noncovalent bonding. The most important step in the synthesis of collagen is the vitamin C–dependent hydroxylation of the proline. It is this step that provides the tensile strength of collagen and, consequently, wound healing. The depletion of vitamin C in sailors led to scurvy and, ultimately, to poor wound healing and loss of dentition in this population. This major step is also inhibited by systemic steroids, thus resulting in poor wound strength and delayed healing. Hyperbaric oxygen also acts at this step, catalyzing the hydroxylation and improving wound strength as well as accelerating healing.

Wound Strength

Wound strength follows a typical curve in an ideal situation (**Fig. 8**). As one can see, the wound strength begins to plateau around 4 to 5 weeks, reaching around 60% of its original strength. Once healed, it reaches its maximum strength (only 80% of its original) at approximately 1 year.[12] This curve has important implications when selecting suture material to primarily close incisions when material such as Vicryl loses the majority of its strength at 1 month. Sutures are used to close gaping wounds, prevent hemorrhage and infection, support wound strength, and provide an aesthetically pleasing result. The major delineations between materials are monofilament versus multifilament and absorbable versus nonabsorbable. The biomaterial characteristics of different suture material and the time for which

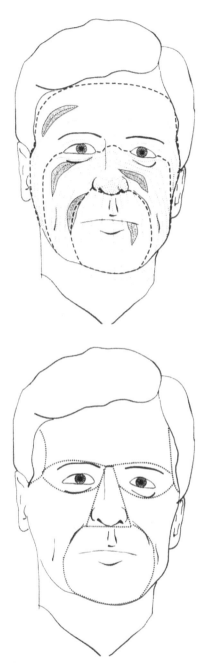

Fig. 7. The relaxed skin tension lines and facial subunit are helpful to plan incisions to achieve optimal appearance of scars. (*Reprinted from* Hom DB, Odland R. Prognosis for facial scarring. In: Harahap M, editor. Surgical techniques for cutaneous scar revision. New York: Marcel Dekker; 2000. p. 31; with permission.)

of this article but they warrant a comprehensive approach for treatment, which obviates the need to monitor surgical wounds. One needs to monitor for the two most common complications, bleeding and infection, using the old tenets of "dolor, rubor,

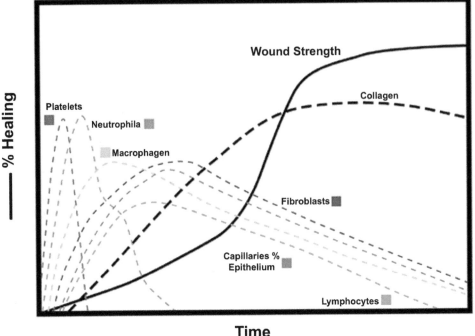

Fig. 8. The typical curve of the increase in wound tensile strength as time progresses. Strength plateaus around 4 to 5 weeks and reaches only 80% of its original strength. (*Reprinted from* emedicine: Wound healing, chronic wounds. Available at: http://emedicine.medscape.com/article/1298452-overview; with permission.)

tensile strength is no longer needed in wound closure is important for choosing the best suture material. One of the basics is the desire to close the wound with suture that will maintain its strength until the wound itself begins to plateau on the tensile curve (4–5 weeks). This time varies—less for mucosal surfaces and more for areas of tension—hence the need for differing suture materials for these areas.

Cytokines in Wound Healing

Cytokines are important signaling molecules that are essential to the healing process. Our current understanding of wound healing has shown the important effects of cytokines; however, most of our knowledge is from in vitro studies. More than 30 cytokines are involved in wound healing produced by macrophages, platelets, fibroblasts, epidermal cells, and neutrophils.[10] Our ability to predict and modify the expression of these cytokines has been much the focus. Future skin scar research is active, especially in the role of transforming growth factor (TGF)-β and the different subtypes that can either impair healing or accelerate healing. The key to the clinical applications of this research will be the cytokine delivery method and the timing of application.

Basic Tenets of Wound Healing

To optimize wound healing there are several basic tenets that one can follow. Winter,[13] in studying epithelialization in pigs, noted 3 critical factors important for the healing of cutaneous wounds:

1. Wound hydration
2. Blood supply
3. Infection minimization.

The ability of ointments and occlusive dressings to trap moisture in the wound has been shown to double the speed of epithelialization.[14] This process prevents desiccation of the upper dermis and allows for more rapid epithelialization. A rolled wound edge is the clinical indicator that epithelialization has been halted. By freshening the wound edge, it helps stimulate and transform the quiescent epithelial cells into migrating keratinocytes to travel over the wound bed. The epithelial layer serves as a physical barrier to prevent infection and desiccation.

Intrinsic and Extrinsic Factors in Wound Healing

Factors affecting wound healing can be divided into intrinsic and extrinsic factors (**Box 1**). Intrinsic

Box 1
A nonexhaustive list of the intrinsic and extrinsic factors that affect healing

Intrinsic factors

- Age
  - Fetus
  - Child
  - Adult
- Immune status
- Hypertrophic scarring and keloids
- Psychophysiological stress
  - Stress
  - Pain
  - Noise
- Hereditary healing diseases
  - Ehlers-Danlos syndrome
  - Epidermolysis bullosa
  - Marfan syndrome
  - Osteogenesis imperfecta
  - Werner syndrome
- Disease states
  - Chronic pulmonary disease
  - Chronic cardiac disease
  - Chronic liver disease (cirrhosis)
  - Uremia
  - Alcoholism
  - Diabetes
  - Peripheral vascular disease

Extrinsic factors

- Malnutrition
  - Protein-calorie
  - Vitamins
  - Minerals
- Infection
- Insufficient oxygenation or perfusion
  - Hypoxemia
  - Hypoxia
  - Anemia
  - Hypovolemia
- Smoking
- Cancer
- Radiation
- Chemotherapy
- Medications
  - Steroids
  - Anticoagulants
  - Penicillamine
  - Cyclosporine

Reprinted from Hom DB, Odland R. Prognosis for facial scarring. In: Harahap M, editor. Surgical techniques for cutaneous scar revision. New York: Marcel Dekker; 2000. p. 25–37; with permission.

factors are those related to the overall health of the patient and any predisposing factors. In general, any connective tissue and inflammatory disorders influence wound healing, such as in any patient with alterations in the key components of wound healing including leukocytes, protein production, and relative or actual immunodeficiencies (human immunodeficiency virus, diabetes, and so forth). Other obvious factors that decrease wound healing are chronic or acute diseased states including liver disease, uremia, malignancy, sepsis, and shock. Patients affected by these conditions may have limited ability to mount an immune response, provide less oxygenation to healing tissues, or have a diminished nutritional supply for the healing process.

AGE IN WOUND HEALING

As we age, our ability to heal decreases as a result of decreased collagen density, fewer fibroblasts, increased elastin fragmentation, and slower wound contraction. Age-related healing was reportedly first studied in World War I by P. Lacompte du Nouy, who noted that it took almost twice as long for a 40-year-old man to close a 40-cm^2 wound than for his 20-year-old compatriot. Although his studies did not involve controls for many variables, it did begin the focus on age-related changes in the skin and their effects on healing.

As we age, the total amount of collagen in the dermis decreases by 1% per year. The epidermal turnover time decreases as well, most dramatically after the age of 50. The dermis also becomes relatively acellular and avascular. These age-related changes, along with the many systemic diseases that occur later in life, all translate into slower and less effective healing.[15]

INFECTION IN WOUND HEALING

Preventing infections in wounds includes debriding necrotic tissue, absorbing exudate, and decreasing bacterial colonization. Bacterial load greater than 10^5 per gram of tissue leads to infection and delayed healing.[16] The goal of wound care is to keep the bacterial load below this critical value, achieved by lightly packing any dead space in the wound and using gentle dressings to most appropriately treat the wound, thus preventing accumulation of any exudates that can be a nidus for infection. Diverting salivary flow is important in preventing exposure of the wound to enzymes and oral flora. The plethora of available wound dressings to prevent infection is out of the purview of this article.

IMMUNE FUNCTION IN WOUND HEALING

Whether alterations to immune function are intrinsic or extrinsic, their effect on the inflammatory phase of healing leads to poor wound healing. Immunosuppressed individuals are less able to fight infection but also lack proper functioning or quantity of inflammatory cells to proper follow the inflammatory phase. If improper cellular debridement of the wound occurs via these cells, wound healing is delayed and ultimately leads to more scarring.

Exogenous use of anti-inflammatory medications can alter the healing environment within the first 3 days of healing. Essential molecular modulators are released within these first 3 days of the inflammatory phase, and any medications that alter this phase will, in turn, alter healing. Corticosteroids, immunosuppressants, or chemotherapy agents are the prime culprits. In practice, it is optimal to have patients off these medications for at least 1 month before surgery and for at least 1 to 2 weeks after surgery. Once the inflammatory phase has concluded, it is less essential to be off these medications.[17]

DIABETES AND WOUND HEALING

Diabetics have poor wound healing for many reasons. Decreased perfusion caused by accelerated atherosclerosis and neuropathy make diabetic patients an increased risk for infection. Along with decreased immune function, this sets up a scenario for prolonged and abnormal healing. Besides the obvious immune dysfunction, diabetics also have slower collagen synthesis and accumulation, decreased angiogenesis, and poorer tensile strength of wounds, leading to higher rate of dehiscence. Tight control of hyperglycemia is essential in the diabetic healing wound, sometimes even necessitating hospitalization and endocrine consultation.

HYPERTROPHIC SCARRING AND KELOIDS

Although keloids are discussed in other articles in this publication (see "Keloids: Prevention and Management" by Sidle and Kim), they deserve mention here for their role in predicting scarring based on patient factors. Hypertrophic scars and keloids are the result of an enhanced proliferative phase of healing and decreased collagen lysis, which are the end result of excessive immature collagen (type III) and especially ECM (water and glycoprotein) deposition. Hypertrophic scars stay within the boundaries of the original wound, whereas keloids extend beyond the limits of the wound. Both entities have been found in all races, but tend to affect darker-pigmented individuals. Of note, keloids have not yet been reported in albinos. African Americans have the highest rate of keloid formation (6%–16%). Although they can occur anywhere, the body areas most susceptible to this abnormal scarring include the earlobe, angle of mandible, upper back and shoulders, upper arms, and anterior chest. Hormonal factors play a role, as they usually are prominent only in women during the fertile years (puberty to menopause). Increased areas of wound tension are also susceptible, thus reiterating the need for tension-free closures. Concern for the development of keloid is in the third week when the proliferative phase appears to continue unabatedly. At this point it is difficult to determine whether keloid or hypertrophic scar will occur and, despite extensive research, it is still undetermined as to what causes the transition from one to the other. TGF-β seems to play a large role in keloid formation, as there is enhanced mRNA expression of TGF-β1 in keloid tissue.[18]

OXYGEN DELIVERY IN WOUND HEALING

Perfusion and oxygenation are the key elements of wound healing and are the two most common reasons for failure of wound healing. Oxygen is key in many steps of the wound-healing process including inflammation, bactericidal activity, angiogenesis, epithelialization, and collagen deposition. Collagenases operate best between oxygen levels of 20 and 200 mm Hg, and human incisions average 30 to 40 mm Hg. Any alterations in the delivery of oxygen, such as vasoconstriction due to hypovolemia, catecholamines, stress, and cold slow the course of wound healing. Wounds of the head and face as well as the anus, compared with extremities, show remarkable healing times because of their high vascularity. Wound Pao_2 can be maximized with increased perfusion and exogenous supplemental oxygen to achieve oxygen levels of 100 mm Hg, which can improve chronic wound healing.[19]

NUTRITION IN WOUND HEALING

Protein and DNA synthesis are essential elements of the healing process. Any diminution of the building blocks (ie, amino acids and nucleic acids) or any cofactors involved in these processes can have detrimental effects on the wound. Malnutrition of any sort can have a strong negative effect but protein deficiency has a profound effect, due to the large amount of collagen synthesis that takes place. A depleted protein status leads to decreased fibroblast proliferation, decreased proteoglycan and collagen synthesis, decreased angiogenesis, and altered collagen remodeling.[6] Albumins of less than 1.5 mg/dL result in poor collagen production and overall poor wound healing.[20] Poor carbohydrate reserve/intake leads to protein catabolism with subsequent depletion of proteins essential to healing. These effects are seen most dramatically in acute malnutrition states (weeks before and after injury). Vitamin deficiencies can also lead to poor healing, especially vitamins C and A, zinc, and thiamine. Vitamin C and thiamine (B1) are essential in collagen formation, and deficiencies lead to decreased cross-linking and, ultimately, wound strength. Vitamin A is essential to the inflammatory process, but its role is not fully understood. Zinc is another cofactor key to wound healing that should be supplemented in the perioperative period, especially in high-risk populations (ie, head and neck cancer). A weight loss of 10% or greater is the general cutoff for severe malnutrition, seen in many of the head and neck cancer patients who require reconstruction. Even a short period of repletive enteral nutrition via nasogastric tube will significantly improve postoperative healing.[21]

SMOKING IN WOUND HEALING

Smoking has long been known to affect the healing process. It is believed that besides the direct toxic effects of the constituents of cigarettes, the most harm results from the generalized vasoconstrictive effects of nicotine. Sorenson and colleagues[22] studied 78 smokers for 15 weeks and divided them into 3 groups. The first group smoked 20 cigarettes a day before and in the weeks following wounding. The next group smoked 20 cigarettes a day before and used a nicotine patch after wounding. The last group was abstinent throughout. The infection rate of the 2 smoking groups was 12% compared with 2% in the nonsmokers. In fact, abstinence for 4 weeks prior to wounding resulted in a dramatic decrease in infection but no change in wound dehiscence. Nonsmokers did not have any wound dehiscence. Smoking has been shown to decrease the function of neutrophils, inhibit collagen synthesis, and increase levels of carboxy-hemoglobin. Interestingly enough, nicotine patch users had no adverse events, which led to the conjecture that other components in cigarette smoke contribute to poor healing. In general, most facial surgeons recommend abstinence from smoking for at least 4 to 6 weeks, if not longer, especially when undertaking elective skin-flap surgery.

RADIATION IN WOUND HEALING

Radiation has multiple effects on wound healing, which can be classified as short-term and long-term effects. Radiation in the short term induces a state of microvascular obliteration and fibrosis, and alters cellular replication.[6] Chronic changes are attributable to the effects on blood vessels, causing narrowing of all vessel sizes and vessel wall degeneration. Optimal timing for surgical procedures in radiation patients should be after the acute injury period but before the chronic phase has taken hold. This period translates to between 3 weeks and 3 months following radiation therapy.[21,23]

CHEMOTHERAPY IN WOUND HEALING

These therapeutic agents are directed at altering cellular replication at multiple levels. The cells most affected are those that undergo rapid turnover. Bone marrow suppression of cells directly involved in the healing process are also affected, which results in fewer monocytes and megakaryocytes, and thus fewer circulating platelets and macrophages. Obvious delays in healing result.

FUTURE RESEARCH IN WOUND HEALING

Much of the recent research in wound healing has been on cytokine and chemokine modulation. Much research has been dedicated to the role of TGF-β and its isomers with their differing effects on healing. TGF-β1 was studied by Zugmaier and colleagues[24] when it was given intraperitoneally to nude mouse models for 10 days; this led to marked fibrosis and scarring. Shah and colleagues[25–27] have studied neutralizing antibodies against profibrotic TGF-β1, with good results, and also studied the role of TGF-β3 and its antifibrotic effects. The critical step in this process is to not only understand the type of cytokines to target but also when to target them to most effectively modulate healing.

Self-Test Responses

The following are correct responses to the self-test presented at the beginning of this article.

1. A 19-year-old woman is on isotretinoin (Accutane) for acne and has a facial acne scar that she wishes to be dermabraded. What do you counsel the patient about?

   Correct answer: She needs to be off the medication for 1 year to limit the risk of scarring

   Incorrect:

   - She should continue the medication because the extra vitamin A will improve her healing.
   - You cannot resurface her acne scar because of the long-lasting effects of this medication.
   - Encourage 2 g of vitamin C daily for 2 weeks before the procedure.

2. A 73-year-old insulin-dependent diabetic man with a serum glucose level of 300 mmol/L comes to your office for a rhytidectomy. How do you optimize your results?

   Correct answer: Refer to endocrinologist for tight diabetic control before surgery

   Incorrect:

   - Decline the surgery because the risk of failure is increased.
   - Start the patient on vitamin E supplementation 2000 IE daily 2 weeks before surgery.
   - Double his insulin dose on the morning of his surgery.

3. A 30-year-old man has a partial-thickness 4 × 4-cm abrasion on his right cheek. What should be the best treatment?

   Correct answer: Keep the wound bed moist with a moisture-retentive ointment

   Incorrect:

   - Place a split-thickness skin graft.
   - Place a full-thickness skin graft.
   - Keep the wound dry to maximize reepithelialization.

4. A 50-year-old man sees you about a large wide scar on his neck. On inquiring, the patient states he had a lymph node removed last year and this scar has grown bigger than the cyst was. What do you counsel him about?

   Correct answer: That this is a keloid and that multiple procedures along with steroid injections may be required to excise it, but still there is no guarantee it will be removed completely

   Incorrect:

   - That he most likely has a hypertrophic scar and that the likelihood is that this will not happen on further surgical procedures.
   - That this is a keloid and that with vitamin E ointments it should resolve.
   - That this is a hypertrophic scar with completely go away with simple excision.

REFERENCES

1. Sipos P, Gyory H, Hagymasi K, et al. Special wound healing methods used in Ancient Egypt and the mythological background. World J Surg 2004;28:211–6.
2. Mogensen M, Morsy HA, Thrane L, et al. Morphology and epidermal thickness of normal skin imaged by optical coherence tomography. Dermatology 2008;217(1):14–20.
3. Ha RY, Nojima K, Adams WP Jr, et al. Analysis of facial skin thickness: defining the relative thickness index. Plast Reconstr Surg 2005;115(6):1769–73.
4. Hom DB. Wound healing in relation to scarring. Facial Plast Surg Clin North Am 1998;6:11.
5. Larouche D, Lavoie A, Germain L, et al. Identification of epithelial stem cells in vivo and in vitro using keratin 19 and BrdU. Methods in Molecular Biology. In: Turksen K, editor, Epidermal cells, vol. 289. Clifton (NJ): Humana Press; 2005. p. 383–400.
6. Hom DB, Odland R. Prognosis for facial scarring. In: Harahap M, editor. Surgical techniques for cutaneous scar revision. New York: Marcel Dekker; 2000. p. 25–37.
7. Rodero M, Khosrotehrani K. Skin wound healing modulation by macrophages. Int J Clin Exp Pathol 2010;3(7):643–53.

8. Robson MC. Proliferative scarring. Surg Clin North Am 2003;83:557–69.

9. Pilcher BK, Wang M, Welgus HG, et al. Role of matrix metalloproteinases and their inhibition in cutaneous wound healing and allergic contact hypersensitivity. Ann N Y Acad Sci 1999;878:12–24.

10. Kujath P, Michelsen A. Wounds—from physiology to wound dressing. Dtsch Arztebl Int 2008;105(13): 239–48.

11. Hom DB, Hebda PA, Gosain AK, et al. Essential tissue healing of the face and neck. Shelton (CT): BC Decker and People's Medical Publishing House; 2009.

12. Franz MG, Kuhn MA, Robson MC, et al. Use of the wound healing trajectory as an outcome determinant for acute wound healing. Wound Repair Regen 2000;8(6):511–6.

13. Winter G. Formation of the scab and the rate of epithelialization of superficial wounds in the skin of young domestic pig. Nature 1962;193:293.

14. Alvarez OM, Mertz PM, Eaglstein WH. The effect of occlusive dressings on collagen synthesis and re-epithelialization in superficial wounds. J Surg Res 1983;35(2):142–8.

15. Fenske NA, Lober CW. Structural and functional changes of normal aging skin. J Am Acad Dermatol 1986;15(4):571–85.

16. Robson MC. Wound infection: a failure of wound healing caused by an imbalance of bacteria. Surg Clin North Am 1997;77:637–50.

17. Stadelmann WK, Digenis AG, Tobin GR. Impediments to wound healing. Am J Surg 1998;176(2A Suppl): 39S–47S.

18. Abdou AG, Maraee AH, Al-Bara AM, et al. Immuno-histochemical Expression of TGF-β1 in Keloids and Hypertrophic Scars. The American Journal of Dermatopathology 2011;33(1):84–91.

19. Schreml S, Szeimies RM, Prantl L, et al. Oxygen in acute and chronic wound healing. Br J Dermatol 2010;163(2):257–68.

20. Otranto M, Souza-Netto I, Aquila MB, et al. Male and female rats with severe protein restriction present delayed wound healing. Appl Physiol Nutr Metab 2009;34(6):1023–31.

21. Payne WG, Naidu DK, Wheeler CK, et al. Wound healing in patients with cancer. Eplasty 2008;8:e9.

22. Sorenson LT, Karlsmark T, Gottrup F. Abstinence from smoking reduces incisional wound infection: a randomized control trial. Ann Surg 2003; 238(1):1–5.

23. Hom DB, Adams GL, Monyak D. Irradiated soft tissue and its management. Otolaryngol Clin North Am 1995;28(5):1003–19.

24. Zugmaier G, Paik S, Wilding G, et al. Transforming growth fact beta-1 induces cachexia and systemic fibrosis without an anti-tumor effect in nude mice. Cancer Res 1991;51:3590–4.

25. Shah M, Foreman D, Ferguson MW. Reduction of scar tissue formation in adult rodent wound healing by manipulation of the growth factor profile. J Cell Biochem 1991;S15F:198.

26. Shah M, Foreman D, Ferguson MW. Control of scarring in adult wounds by neutralizing antibody to transforming growth factor β. Lancet 1992;339: 213–4.

27. Shah M, Foreman D, Ferguson MW. Neutralization of TGFB-1 and TGFB-2 or exogenous edition of TGFB-3 to cutaneous rat wounds reduces scarring. J Cell Sci 1995;108:985.

Index

Note: Page numbers of article titles are in **boldface** type.

A

Advanced glycation end products. See
  AGE-products.
Age, wound healing and, 93
AGE-products, action on human skin fibroblasts, 3–4
  in tissue aging, 3–4
  production of, 7
Alginate, as dressing for skin graft donor site, 82
Anodic aluminum oxide, tissue engineering and, 27

B

Basal cell carcinoma, recurrent, full-thickness
  calvarial excision in, with grafting and/or dermal
  substitute, case report of, 65–67
Bone structures, exposed in wounds, skin grafts and
  artificial dermis for management of, **69–75**
Burns, dermal substitutes in, 35–37
  epidermal substitutes in, 35
  tissue engineering in, clinical case of, 28, 29
  total body surface area, autologous split skin
    grafts in, 34–35

C

Calvarial defects, full-thickness, reconstruction of,
  dermal substitutes and split skin grafting with
  artificial dermis in, **65–67**
Candida albicans, 49–50
Cells, functions of, cytoskeletal changes and, 18
  loss of, 1–3
  mechanical properties of, aging and, 9
  viscoelastic properties of, aging and, optical
    stretcher to assess, 12
    and cytoskeletal polymers, and actin, 10
Chemotherapy, in wound healing, 95
Clot formation, skin and, 24
Collagen, in wound healing, 91
Collagen fibers, cross-linking of, age-dependent
  increase in, 3–4
Collagen gels, fibroblast-populated, jasplakinolide in
  treatment of, 16, 17
    rheological properties o, 15–16, 17
    storage and loss of, actin cytoskeleton of cells
      and, 16
Connective tissue, dermis as, 23
Cytokines, in wound healing, 92
Cytoskeletal polymers, and viscoelastic properties
  of cells, 10
Cytoskeleton, actin, of cells, storage and loss of
  fibroblast-populated collagen gels and, 16

as source of mechanical activity of fibroblasts, 15
microtubule, age-related changes in, 14, 16

D

Dermal constructs, commercially available, for
  clinical use, 38–39
Dermal-epidermal junction, harvesting cells from, 26
Dermal substitutes, do well on dura, split skin grafting
  with artificial dermis, for reconstruction of
  full-thickness calvarial defects, **65–67**
Dermal substitutes, in burns, 35–37
Dermatome, powered, in split skin graft, 81
Dermis, appendages of, 87
  as connective tissue, 23
Diabetes, wound healing and, 94

E

Elastase-type endopeptidase activity, increase with
  age, 3
Elastin peptides, elastin receptor for, in aging, 4, 5
  increase in elastase-type activity of fibroblasts
    with, 5, 6
Elastin receptor, for elastin peptides, in aging, 4, 5
Endopeptidase activity, increase in skin fibroblasts,
  with AGE-products, 3–4, 5
Epidermal constructs, commercially available for
  clinical use, 36
Epidermal/dermal substitutes, commercially
  available for clinical use, 37, 40
Epidermal substitutes, in burns, 35
Epidermis, appendages of, 87
European Center for the Validation of Alternative
  Methods, 43
European program for the Registration, Evaluation,
  Authorization and Restriction of Chemicals
  (REACH), 43
Extracellular matrix, and fibroblasts, interaction
  between, 10
    response in healing process, 24
    homeostasis of, cell functions and, 9
    increased degradation of, 3
    loss of, 1
Extracellular matrix scaffold, 25

F

Facial tension lines, to plan incisions, 91
FACS analysis, of human dermal fibroblasts,
  11–12, 14

Printed and bound by CPI Group (UK) Ltd, Croydon, CR0 4YY

03/10/2024

01040356-0003